Leading Prima Care

Resilience

Team Culture

Innovation

Dr Craig Newman

Copyright 2021 © Craig Newman.
Version 1 Published December, 2021
All rights reserved. No part of this publication may be reproduced, stored in a retrieval system, or transmitted, in any form or by any means, electronic, mechanical, photocopying, recording or otherwise, without the prior written permission of the copyright holders.

www.aimyourteam.com

Acknowledgements

Thanks to the primary care teams who inspire this work and the developing leaders who showed me what to share.

Contents

Foreword 2
Introduction 3
1. "We don't have the time" to team build. 6
2. Wellbeing and resilience: the basics 10
3. Key concept for developing leaders. 13

Personal Resilience & Wellbeing 20
4. Self-*ish*-ness: the antidote to burnout in you and your team. 21
5. Working 9 'til 5, what a way to make a living! 27
6. Emotional intelligence as a leader 31
7. How to leave work at work 40
8. Four key needs of compassionate leaders 44
9. Embracing safe uncertainty 50

Leading Primary Care 54
10. Feeling valued as a practice manager 55
11. Feeling valued as a partner GP 62
12. Spend your time most effectively 68
13. Why and how to say 'no', whilst building cohesive teams .. 74
14. The skill and psychology of delegation 78
15. Navigating the partnership boardroom 81

Leading Practice Innovation 86
16. Innovating under pressure 87

17. Winning with large scale innovation 93
18. A game changing skill: process mapping............................103
19. Making change happen: the 30-day plan 107

Team Resilience & Wellbeing 113
20. Sourcing team wellbeing from the team. 114
21. Essential team conversations. 119
22. How much teambuilding time do you need?.......................123
23. Four steps to increase your practice successes 129
24. Check-ins and why they an obvious must............................133
25. Energising and leading an exhausted or disengaged team 139
26. Create capacity through team optimisation.........................143

Summary...148
About the Author 151

Foreword

Welcome to my little book on primary care leadership, through the lens of clinical and organisational psychology, and team coaching theories, approaches and experience.

I claim no lived experience of Primary Care leadership, but the lived experience of supporting many primary care teams and leaders out of a pickle and into sustainable team and leadership being. It is this learning, which is really a privilege to have witnessed, I have decided to spread through the medium of a book.

In all my writing, I hope to convey that I respect your expertise in your own role and hope that you take my insights as ideas and not directives. My intent is never to patronise and always to share insights that might help, this being the core of my occupation and driver in most of my work.

I truly hope engagement with this book provides you some benefit.

Introduction

This book is aimed at providing leaders in Primary Care (Practice Managers and GPs) with thought provoking ideas and approaches that I have seen to positively impact practices in the UK, whilst also being informed by evidence in the broader systemic and wellbeing literatures.

I have written this in the context of a surge in stress, burnout and mental health reports in Primary Care. Whilst many proposed solutions are offered at the level of technological innovation and individual staff wellbeing, this book represents an attempt to support leaders in their own wellbeing, leadership approach, change management and team activation.

There is a huge amount of data emerging which relates to the value of safe teams and change capable teams, but much of this is difficult to translate into primary care teams which are characterised by an unusual business model and often low capacity in the context of very high demand.

In this book I will attempt to acknowledge this context whilst building on skills you already have, an understanding of your challenges, approaches I have seen work and your ability to choose. A light approach to a Psychologically informed body of work, with practices just like yours and people with roles like yours.

How to read this book

This book is a collection of purposefully short stand-alone reads that offer a challenge to problematic thinking and ideas on how to move forwards.

When I refer to problematic thinking, I am referring to beliefs and patterns of coping that get primary care leaders and teams stuck. These thinking styles and associated organisational behaviours can emerge from lengthy NHS service, crippling demand with low capacity, a lack of opportunity to develop leadership skills and, most likely, the complex organisation structure that is a Primary Care practice – a hybrid of NHS service and private business.

This book is a positively intended disruptor for managers and GPs, representing sparks of learning I have observed in supporting practices at the level of individuals, practices and at whole regional networks. Through working with change programmes, accelerators, team coaching and 1 to 1 psychological support, I have witnessed patterns of new thinking and approach that ease the experience of primary care leadership and support teams and leaders to succeed, even in extreme circumstances.

Each section of the book has been designed to be a short read (5 to 7 minutes) and the language is intentionally conversational. This is in recognition of the time pressures staff are under and to force me as a writer to make these ideas simple and accessible. Psychologists can say in 1,000 words what others can say in 100 and primary care staff have only the time to say in 10. I've aimed for a coffee break read that provides a tangible insight and idea each time.

There are four primary themes in the book:

- Personal resilience and wellbeing (for you)
- Leading in Primary Care
- Leading Innovation
- Your team's resilience and wellbeing

The book can be read cover to cover, or you can jump to themes and chapters that stand out as important for you, right now. Although, I do encourage a full read over time. Concepts in the book overlap and ideas call on solutions which are detailed in full in other sections. I try to state where other chapters overlap, to support your wider reading.

Be playful

These are ideas that I encourage you to play with, with your practice team(s). They are not absolute answers and not beyond adaptation by you, to fit your own culture and practice. The key word here is 'play' and I encourage you to lean into ideas that irritate you the most, as these are most likely touching on a raw nerve. Psychologists press harder into such areas and so, without me present with you, I invite you to look out for this and to try the same for yourself.

Take what you need

Play lightly

1. "We don't have the time" to team build.

Increasingly, mental health professionals are receiving referrals from Primary Care for staff support, at the level of the leaders and the team. This will be of no surprise to you, I suspect. I am frequently fielding queries about employee assistant programmes (EAPs) for PCNs, being asked to advise on the best mental health support packages for staff.

I often stun Primary Care leads when I ask, "what are you doing for your teams to make work better and to avoid the need for mental health services, later?".

For many the concept seems foreign or just impossible in the context of barely any time to function, staffing issues and massive demand on services.

I am regularly told, "there isn't any time to work on team building".

Not enough time.

I am pretty much deaf to this phrase. In my work with 100s of teams and 1,000s of individuals, the number one rationale for not improving life and work is the absence of time.

The reason I am deaf to these words is because of my experience of primary care leaders who prioritise team wellbeing, functioning and their own wellbeing but have the same number of hours per day as everyone else. In fact, most surprisingly to new clients, these same leaders usually spend less time at work and so choose to limit the time they have available to get work done.

Having no time is a perception and not a reality for most teams, a truth that is often hard to believe. I realise some teams lose staff and are starting at a low point, but even in this context—a different perspective on capacity is needed.

Team functioning is synonymous with team capacity

This book will drive hard on a message that capacity and team function are synonymous. The better the wellbeing, engagement, unity, and leadership in your practice—for you and your team—the more your team will achieve and succeed in, with less time (more on this in chapter 26).

In this chapter, I want to introduce just a small number of ways team investment is conceptualised within this book, to attack ideas about not enough capacity, head on.

Most of these are detailed with examples in the book:

- *micro appreciations*—noticing and commenting on success in the moment, with team members. Encouraging a culture of this.
- *role clarity*—working on loop to make sure roles are clear and team members are engaged and supported in delivering them.
- *future orientation* — maintaining as positive future success narrative with the team, to support innovation and feelings of safety through crisis.

- *culture shaping*—learning to spot what works well, what the team want more of and committing as a team to creating it.
- *space to think (leaders and team)*—spaces for the leaders and team to reflect on successes and failures, to spark strategic intelligence in place of knee jerk firefighting.
- *check-ins*—small meeting components that can transform engagement and create team awareness of individual needs.
- *'Enabling' 1 to 1s*—using time with staff to invite understanding of their needs and enabling support from you as a leader.
- *team workshops*—intentional spaces for teams to meet who want to accelerate better relationships and engagement.
- *system support*—board level decisions to invest in the team, to ringfence time and to recognise that a positive work environment is economically sensible.

Leaders often don't realise that organisational development and culture design drastically reduces burnout, retention issues, stress, team fractures and illness. This is because individuals start to work together whilst also feeling that being at work is a reward in and of itself, a feeling of being a part of something bigger and greater—where people are in it together. When individual burnout is treated, without organisational change, the effects are often very short (reported at 1 month in some cases, before staff are in need again).

Leaders also don't realise how small actions can be to create huge and positive changes.

It will take a bit of a leap of faith if your team are buried under demand—but the evidence shows that happier teams are protective and engaged teams get more done. The cost of staff retention issues or a GP / practice manager on sick leave for 6 months, due to burnout, is a LOT more than the costs required to address organisational culture and team development.

Team development and culture design can often be fun and rewarding, bringing teams together around a shared mission, something that has never been said about stress related sick leave!

Summary

It is important to hold in mind as you consider team investment, that I regularly refer to small changes and behaviour changes – rather than huge capacity investments. I will propose ideas that require time for your team to work together and these are well worth considering. Teams who are fixed in the belief that there is no time to consider a space to develop together, should not reject the idea of team building entirely. Rather, draw what you can from the ideas in this book that fit into what is available.

There is a leap of faith required to trust the idea that time out with your team will create more capacity. Starting small can help you to build this faith.

Reframe Capacity

Invest into the team

Win Capacity back

2. Wellbeing and resilience: the basics

The basics of wellbeing and resilience are *common knowledge,* but it can take a small nudge to raise awareness of them, when our heads are down working hard.

I'd feel like I was teaching you to suck eggs, if it wasn't for the fact that these themes surface so often with practice leaders that I support. So here are some soft nudges and pointers for you to address as a requirement in being a well and sustainable leader in primary care.

Diet

Are you happy with your diet? If not, why not?

What small improvement could you make this week to shift the dial by 5% towards a better diet?

Commit to this. Review next week and shift the dial 5% more.

Exercise

Do you exercise enough? Exercise creates energy, which all Primary Care clinicians will tell you. Where in your work life could you move a little bit more, just 5% more a day? Start small. Park further away, walk at lunchtime etc. Where in your time outside work can you exercise a little more?

Commit to 2 small actions. Review in 1 week.

Breaks

Do you take breaks and lunch at work? If not, why not?

If your answer is "I don't have time". Read this book and then come back here to answer this question with more insight. Breaks are essential—not a luxury (start with Chapter 5, if this is a recognised priority)

How can you access this essential human need, in your workday? I don't recommend starting small—book off 30 minutes for lunch in your diary and block it out every day. Job done!

Sleep

How is sleep? Do you sleep enough or does work / stress / thinking get in the way? Read about work limits and leaving work at work (debrief), in this book as both as these will help with sleep.

Google search for 'Sleep Hygiene' and follow the rules laid out.

As a Neuro-Psychologist, sleep hygiene and work debriefing were perhaps my two most effective interventions with people who did not sleep well in the context of high pressure work. It is not rocket science, but it takes commitment to the method.

Fun

What is your weekly diet of fun at home AND at work? If you fall short, time to get creative—your mood and energy are related to your access to fun.

Your team can help you create this, you just need to create the spaces to enable it for you all. More on this in the book.

Summary

Simple ideas that are so very true and well evidenced. I have just nudged you to them here, as it can feel very patronising to have this taught to us.

That said, this needs to be read as a minimum requirement, a prescription of a sort. Like all prescriptions, it needs a regular review – so check in monthly on these areas of need. Prolonged compromising on any of these (for you or your team) will lead to unsustainable outcomes or worse.

Audit Needs

Meet Needs

3. Key concept for developing leaders.

Growing up feels so easy to do, it just happens automatically. We learn to walk, interact, speak, run, play, work and much more. A predisposition to absorb and adapt at pace.

It's all neurologically based of course. I say this not to add a dazzling science component to my argument, but to recognise that our drive for novelty and surprise is hard-wired into us. As children, we play and within learning, we experience repeated 'aha' moments that feel pleasurable and fun. Driving us to do more of the same.

Our perception of the world drastically shifts as we age and develop at a neurological level. At one point in time, we couldn't perceive any object existing when it left our sight (object impermanence), but now we realise that the world is more than just what we experience (I hope you do!). At another time, we could not empathise with the complex multi-positional perspective our parents took on our teenage angst, but in later life, we empathise and often feel pity for our poor parents for enduring us.

We grow and shift, but rarely do we notice.

Similar, we don't notice when this process slows to a grinding halt!

Play is replaced with work. Being is replaced with doing. Our lives become littered with deadlines, tasks and goals. We become schooled in rules, performance and outcomes which are many miles away from creative play and innate insight. The relief of meeting a deadline is a poor replacement for the spark of neurological serotonin release that we experience when we truly feel new insight or an epiphany.

In our world of to-do lists and aspirational careers—we don't even notice that growing has become coping.

Coping

We are amazing creatures, us humans. Our psychology and neurology are littered with adaptive processes that can aid us in enduring almost any reality. We learn to repeat what works and to ditch was doesn't. We learn to focus on what feels right and to keep attention away from what irritates or invalidates us. We can tune-up as an unbelievably capable instrument in a particular space, but in doing so—lose sight of how to bounce out of this space and invite new growth on a regular basis.

We cope and coping can be a successful approach.

But the problem with coping is that for most of us, we lean on it far too much, too often and too deeply. We lean on our strengths and shy away from our edges that feel anxiety-provoking, exhausting or confusing. We do this whether our coping skills are functional or dysfunctional.

My work as a therapist and a coach has revealed how very deeply dysfunctional coping strategies can be maintained despite ruining our lives:

- beliefs that we need to just work harder
- beliefs that we must be right, or we are stupid
- beliefs that we are imposters
- beliefs that when things go wrong, it is because we are failures
- beliefs that failure is not acceptable

The list is very long, we all carry them.

Growth

Most of the people I've met have not heard of ideas that the development of our Psychology continues as adults. That we have stages that we can reach, which continue the journey of our development towards more complex thinking, freedom from poor coping strategies and opportunities to feel and be happier.

Most of the people I've met, even if they have heard of this idea or subscribe to it, have not conceived of why it is so difficult for us or why we can get stuck for most of our lives in stages that focus on rules, performance, and goals.

Growth feels different from coping. It feels like a continued experience of 'Aha' moments, with release from old pressures and an expanded feeling of just getting what it's all about.

This sounds quite vague I realise. But when I've witnessed clients experience it, and my own experience of it—it is so hard to articulate. Clients say things like, "I feel lighter" and "I just didn't know this before" and "it kind of makes sense in a way I can't speak".

Just like object permanence arrived as toddlers who realise objects exist when not seen, new insights arrive as adults—but it is so very hard to notice this and to draw comparisons to an older version of our mind that now feels distant and less in touch.

For almost everyone I've supported, who has seen improvement, some form of growth occurred.

This includes patients I have worked with facing death in their 20s or 30s, recovering from illness and injuries or in tremendous permanent pain.

It also includes leaders and teams who have endured fatigue, stress and a sense of being in over their heads—to emerge calm, collected and serene. It is a human commonality and so seen in many spaces when stimulated.

Stimulating Growth

Humans have the innate capacity and desire to grow—to expand psychologically. I know this and feel it, I've seen it in 1,000s of people in all walks of life.

We also have every ingredient to get in the way of this.

- unfinished business in our past that irritates us and sabotages us now
- roles and tasks that don't invite play
- a doing approach rather than a reflective approach

- a lack of understanding on how to 'think' creatively to grow (supported by our education system's approach to learning)
- environments that pull us towards goals and don't invite space to think

We can grow and adapt beyond these states of being, with the right roadmap, and much of this is touched on by the sections and the chapters that are to follow…

A blended approach is needed in which we work towards a great insight into our past and why we have reached a dead-end in growth. This has to be paired with priming our environment to support our change, whilst also aiming our energy and efforts at growing the context of the challenges we already face. We don't need new challenges, we just need to transform the ones we have from coping to transformation opportunities.

The last is developing compassionate and reflective thinking styles and spaces that in many ways echo the play and creativity of our childlike minds—but again, aimed at growth where we need it (more on this in chapter 8)

It is incredibly difficult to take this journey alone, although not impossible. I'd argue that when you feel exhausted, struggling to balance life and work or a sense of loss of control/disillusionment—you can get the best gains from being supported.

As a most simple primer on growth, I'd advise:

INSIGHTS

- consider your past and look for repeated self-sabotage/patterns of struggle. Tell your own story and know it.
- consider what pain points in your life echo most often in your life and consider how stubborn they are. They may need to be wobbled out of your way.

LEANING INTO GROWTH

- create space in your environment to be strategic and reflective—an adult version of play at work.
- aim your growth at what you need, not at solving a problem. e.g. I need to be more in control of what energy I spend on work tasks, I need to calibrate consciously etc.
- Be self-compassionate.

REFLECT / INVITE GROWTH

- invite a reflective practice on a regular basis
- reflect on your own growth to spark 'Aha' moments
- play with ideas and expect to fail often…
- …reframe failure as learning!

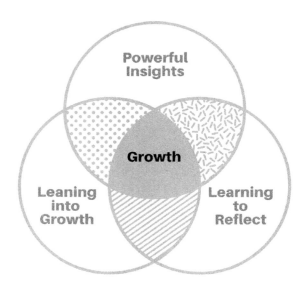

Our 3 pillars approach to stimulating growth, the 'aimyourteam growth' model.

Take this same approach at the level of your team and board. Create insight of areas that need to change, lean into these as a team and expect to learn through failure. Realise that without this playful approach, we often get stuck or fail to learn as we try to adapt.

Pause

Breath

Play

Personal Resilience & Wellbeing

"Don't confuse having a career with having a life"

Hilary Clinton

4. Self-*ish*-ness: the antidote to burnout in you and your team.

It is my observation that the public sector is riddled with rescuers. People who put the needs of others first. This is perhaps the core superpower of the public sector!

This is true in Primary Care, where services are drowning in demand and the outcome is often burnt-out staff across the whole team.

In this chapter we will consider what amount we should give to others and what amount we should be giving to ourselves and our team.

Unsustainable giving

Increasingly, in my supportive role alongside primary care—whether it is compassion, empathy, work effort, task performance or any other role metric being referred to, the word fatigue is now regularly attached to it.

   Compassion fatigue
   Work fatigue
   Performance fatigue
   Innovation fatigue
   Digital fatigue

One thing is now very clear, if it wasn't already, that it is unsustainable to give excessive amounts of ourselves away, without much in return. In the context of this unsustainability, the word "burnout" is also increasingly used.

Burnout and fatigue are risk factors in healthcare, not only for the person but also in terms of patients outcomes. The cruel twist here is that the harder teams work to meet patient needs, the more risk they introduce that they will fail to meet them or make serious errors.

It is hard to see whilst in it, but a constant barrage of demand, daily firefighting and suffocating in tasks - breaks staff, fractures teams and puts patients at risk.

None of this is new for you to hear, I suspect.

What to do about it?

Limits on giving

Little can be done, in any immediate timeframe, on the demands placed on Primary Care. Certainly, at the level of an individual practice.

One of the things that teams and the people within them can do is to draw a line on what a team can sustainably give. There are times, for all teams, where giving our all is needed and leaders rally teams at these times. But there is really no rational way to hold this rally call indefinitely—and although it seems a solution and perhaps the only one at hand, staff will become ill, people will quit and many of those who don't will likely burnout, become difficult to manage and at risk in their role.

To make the idea of giving and receiving more tangible, I often ask primary care leaders the question—how percentage of yourself do you give to others every day, in your role? Your energy, capacity, drive, time…

Many, many leaders in Primary Care give me absolute replies such as, "all of myself" or high figures such as "80-95%".

What would be your answer to this question?

Pause and answer this question now.

I suspect the answer is high.

I propose to staff that their answer should never exceed 51% and this is a maximum, not an ideal, so should perhaps be lower.

This is usually met with a laugh or swear word as my client considers that I know nothing about the realities of their job.

It is true that I can only infer what it is to be a practice manager or GP, but I can also infer what it means to not cope in both roles—having worked with many, many of your colleagues who can't go on. All of these staff gave similar high number responses and all of them could not sustain it.

Recharging at work

Work can have many sources of recharge and positivity:

- feeling valued
- status
- balance
- choice
- control
- achievement
- personal development
- team unity

All of these can be built into primary care roles to make it *feel* like staff are receiving and not just giving. Notice now, most of these relate to our experience of work with our team, with other people or with our organisation, rather than the specific tasks we are performing.

It is an error to think that I am talking about amounts of time when I talk about percentages of giving of yourself, as I am not. Rather, I am referring to whether a task feels like a drain or a recharge.

For example, time with a team can be exhausting or it can feel like a teaming up with our supporters. Time in clinic can feel isolated and overwhelming, or rewarding when you are in control of your lists and feeling a shared load with other clinicians. Difficult work challenges can be balanced by a sense of being truly valued and being invested in by the practice, to develop upwards. Time as a leader can feel riddled with fear about the future or like a regular stride in a confident persona.

51% of work tasks (or more!) need to be nurturing and recharging—any less and we are in slow depletion towards zero, if sustained.

Self-ish-ness

In our culture we see selfishness as a negative. This is even worse in public sector workers, in my experience. Who regularly put themselves last in the throes of work.

Being selfish is a powerful antidote to burnout and stress.

Accepting that the word selfish simply means, a bit of yourself in your thinking, is helpful to us. The word is created by joining self and *ish*, the ish meaning a little bit. In fact, once you realise that the word simply infers a little bit of yourself in your thinking about your world, you will also realise it is crazy that we reject the word so much. The alternative is to be zero self, as selfish is just a little bit away from that.

Surely you can't argue for zero self as an ideal for you and your team?

Selfishness should be promoted in all staff. This is through a culture of conversations, reflection, listening, task design and openness (all covered in this book). We build sustainable and engaged experiences of work by topping up the tank of everyone at work—a 51% recharge to the 49% depletion hard line in the sand.

It is a mind shift that is critical—more so in current times.

Summary

Creating a narrative that people need their needs, desires and drives met from at least 51% of their work activity, is the goal for teams. Make this a team value alongside patient care, as patient care cannot be sustained without it.

This is not about working less—but about changing the meaning and shared experience of work.

This book is full of ideas to help with this—but here, we set the limits you should be aiming at. The higher the figure, above 51%, the happier you and your team!

Ask

Notice Needs

Meet Needs

5. Working 9 'til 5, what a way to make a living!

Dolly Parton clearly did not work in Primary Care.

"The idea of 9 to 5 is impossible, intangible and for a reality for everyone else outside of the NHS."

After two decades in the NHS, I accept that 9 to 5 is a stretch of the imagination to make reality for many staff. However, my experience of Primary Care leaders is that you can get quite close to this if you optimise your team and set your values up in a way that protect you and them.

This idea creates a lot of resistance in many Primary Care leaders when I meet them and talk about it. That said, most over workers don't like the way they are working and the impact on their lives. Weekends are about recovery and holidays are a quarter stress detox as work is dropped behind followed by a quarter stress revving up, on the way back in.

If asked, when you were a teen, what do you want to be when you get older—I doubt you'd have replied with, "working 12-hour days, some weekends, exhausted and most of that unpaid overtime".

Holding up this mirror can create anger and I might be wrong in terms of some of the facts, but I risk this response when I challenge primary care leaders who tell me there is no choice in the way they work —as people get lost in their own narratives. Managers and GPs often tell me this is the reality of primary care, unaware that others I have worked with have a counter narrative and work with a greater life balance. They have taken a journey away from this sense of reality to creating something new and more sustainable.

Where to start

It starts with believing that a life balance is possible and setting it as a concrete value in your team. A value you want for yourself, for them and a value they want for you.

Perhaps 8 to 6 is your compromise, and I've met many who have chosen this. Within this, I'd be asking what breaks you take and where you have lunch and with who.

Lunch!?!?

Yes, your younger self probably expected you to eat during the day too and to perhaps take a break or two.

It is a difficult concept to grasp, but when we don't set limits around when we are at work, or not, we create a need for us to be there. Enablement of a sort. When we respond to emails and texts at 6am or 10pm, we create the demand or we perceive the demand.

If I open a shoe shop from 7am until 10pm, I will get customers all day long. I might then assume I have to stay open to meet demand, but in reality, if I close at 5pm (like all other shoe shops) the customers come earlier. But it can be hard to make this choice, as we feel a risk that we will lost that rare 9.55pm customer who wants the most expensive shoes on the shelf.

When we save up work to take home, we gift ourselves more time to do it. We don't force ourselves to be creative, to say no more often, to focus our role, to focus the team, to use the team and to spend time wisely. The larger the pot of resource, the more we drink from it. Unfortunately, it is us who must refill it and when we don't get energy back from life, it drains quickly.

Believe it or not, other GPs and Practice managers do go home on time, stay away from work at home and come back the next day refreshed. I've met some of them and even facilitated a few to become this. Perhaps not the norm, but trailblazers who have created a trail worth following them down.

Reframe the problem to activate your strengths

This is a very brief chapter that aims at disrupting your belief in time and work.

What do you want? 6–7, 7–6, 8–6, 9–6 or (dare I say it) 9–5?

Write it down and shrink your diary to your desire.

Then you have a new problem- rather than how to get more time you now have to make it work within time boundaries. And guess what, primary care leads are EXCEPTIONAL at solving resource problems, arguably the best in the world! Once you make this a real problem to solve and you use the whole team to do it (more on this later in this book), you will be amazed at how you can.

Summary

Those of you who work too long and don't like it—you perhaps just haven't aimed yourself yet at being tough on time and brilliant at solving the problems this brings.

Time to make that change?

Set limits

Feel the pain

Solve the pain

6. Emotional intelligence as a leader

I'm pretty sure that Gorden Gecko (Wall Street) was not correct when he said, "lunch is for wimps" — but his inference that those who want success don't take lunch seems right, in the minds of many leaders.

This seems especially true in the minds of Primary Care leaders I have met. I regularly hear leaders telling me that they work through lunch, don't take breaks and face an ever-increasing workload in the context of accelerating change and an uncertain future.

It is tempting to say, "take lunch" or "take breaks"(as I did in the last chapter) — but this will likely irritate the psychological drivers that cause us to put ourselves last and in to overdrive. Whilst we do need pace and breaks, we also need to understand and sooth the emotions that create these patterns of working.

Here I will offer some psychological insight, on why self-sacrifice and relentless work has become the norm — and what to do about it.

Me, myself & threat

When I watch our neighbour's dog lying on his blanket out in the sun, I often envy the contentment he can so easily access. When a car passes or our cat emerges, his calm instantly switches into a frenzied state where he shouts for all to hear and races with all of his might at his new target. I hear him enter this state many times in the day and similarly see him lying there, deep in slumber.

Much of his neurological anatomy, we as humans share. We carry the same adrenal system that can at any moment spot a threat or exciting stimuli and kick into gear. In an instant, we can go from calm to fully activated both physically and neurologically. Physically designed through evolution to fight or fly, to access our full potential in an instant.

Much is known about our adrenal response. Both that for a time it improves our functioning both physically and mentally. In fact, as humans we perform better for a time if we are stressed — hence the need for goals and performance orientation as leaders and teams.

But if activated for too long we slide into exhaustion and eventual burnout.

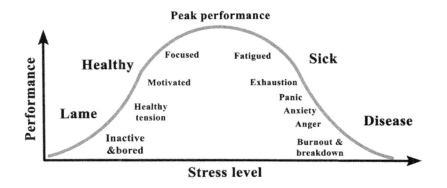

Unlike my neighbour's dog, our psychology is equipped with a rich tapestry of additional psychological capabilities than enable us to live and succeed but can become the drivers rather than our support mechanisms. The performance curve is shown above — a neurological fail-safe to enable us to fight external threats, can in fact be driven by internal threats. Our own thoughts.

When the threat is inside us and the outcome is to fight or run away — which we can't, we can become locked in a cycle where doing feels like resolving. There are a great amount of psychological coping strategies and concepts at play in the context of rapid change, uncertainty, increased pressure and perceived threat. The context many leaders like you are in right now.

To offer a succinct summary, consider us as meaning-making machines. Our neurology has to somehow marry up a biological response and survival system with both external and internal (often imagined) threats.

We have lots of clever ways of doing this including avoidance, noticing only the things that confirm what we want to see (confirmation bias), a preference for familiarity (familiarity bias), an ability to see certainty in the context of uncertainty (existentialism) and a surge to act in response to threat (fight or flight)… and more.

Put together — in the right context — and we have a Molotov cocktail that can create a wildfire of activity that burns up all of our energy with a thick smoke that masks our ability to think beyond putting out fires.

We surge to act, which feels like responding to threat. We create or imagine certainty in the context of uncertainty, spending huge amounts of psychological energy persuading ourselves that we have control over all events and trying to pass this on to our teams. We rely more on what we have seen work well in the past, as change and newness threaten our state of certainty — which reduces our ability to innovate well. We fail to see or hear new ideas or even our own inner voice, as we seek to confirm and reinforce the state of solid ground, we feel ourselves creating. Our actions show us we are responding, which offers some comfort — but the adrenal system does not abate as our inner psychology rages and we push hard on our coping systems to ignore it.

Add into this the pressure of demand outstripping capacity, staff issues, clinical crises, and rapid constant change directives — and our Molotov cocktail just became napalm. Our response, we fix in an escalating loop of doing more and resting less.

Sounds tiring.

It is and it seems very common in primary care, at varying degrees.

Soothing your psychological response

I rarely hear primary care leaders talks about soothing or self-compassion, there are some whispers about these ideas but it is a shy story amongst a much louder story of what leaders can 'do'.

I argue that leaders need to educate and expand their capacity for intentionally being, intentionally activating states of emotion that calm their being, managing energy expenditure and activating psychological perceptions that enable a mediated relationship with their work and consequential psychological response.

Less is sometimes more… a cliche I hope to persuade you is true when it comes to 'doing'.

Things to consider:

Validate your own emotions

It is important to realise that we bring our whole selves to work. I hear this parroted to me by leaders all of the time, often when they are talking about their team. But as leaders, we carry our emotions at work and we either listen to the disruptive emotions and soothe them, else we project them into our work and team.

A leader who is fearful of failure and lets this run wild will project all sorts of behaviours at the team to create a safety net for themselves or to pass the emotions off as they are just too big to hold. Anger, stress, fatigue, resentment, overwhelm – they are all potential small bombs that get in the way of functioning teamwork.

It is important to be available for yourself and the emotions you are carrying. They are not your enemy; they are your needs made felt emotions. Many leaders tell me they fear dumping their emotions onto their teams — but this is more likely if you don't attend to them. This is not an all or nothing suggestion. You can feel sometimes, show a little vulnerability and be human. The bigger stuff, reflect on.

Reflect

I often ask clinical leaders how much thinking they expect or hope from the likes of Boris Johnson (PM, 2021) or Amanda Pritchard (NHS CEO, 2021). How much doing and how much thinking in a given day?

Ask yourself this (try not to be sarcastic!).

I am told that people really hope both are thinking a lot. Which infers that they must be stopping their 'doing' to actually spend time 'thinking'.

It's a leading question of course, as I then ask — how much thinking would your practice team hope you are doing, as the leader?

How much are you actually doing?
How much time do you ringfence for thinking — not talking and planning with others, but sitting, strategising, reflecting on your leadership and allowing your feelings to be data for your leadership?

It is not rocket science to see how this might help — but beyond this feeling intuitive, note that reflection is a core of almost every executive coaching programme and clinical therapy model. It is seen as central to personal growth, coping and leadership success.

Growth and learning are built on a foundation of being able to observe yourself in action, from a position of reflection. It might interest you to know that research has shown that this type of reflective practice increased both energy and engagement for leaders alongside similar testimonials from my own clients – leaders and teams.

Calibrate

We can often think that reflection is a type of thinking, whereas it is important to also consider it as a type of listening to what we feel.

What emotions are we feeling and what is our body feeling. Do we feel charged up, drained, aching, tense and where in our bodies do we feel this? How often do we notice this and should we try to notice it more?

Calibration is learning to be intentional about what state we are in, based on what the tasks or context need. We may have fallen into a pattern of supercharged performance and alertness for the whole day, but perhaps we only really need this for an hour. Perhaps our emails and admin need us to down gear, to drop energy expenditure and see these tasks as a physical break from fight or flight — a kind of slow lap around the track to help us get our breath back.

Learning to calibrate and to model this to our teams — is a crucial step towards creating optimal performance in a culture that also supports recovery.

Embrace safe uncertainty

In a world of obvious uncertainty and change, you need to equip yourself to know the answer enough to feel safe. This may sound contradictory — how can we know what we don't know?

The truth is, we always did.

We drive past car crashes without any shift in our sense of how safe we are in our own cars. We live in an uncertain world and are very experienced in not letting it derail us.

We have developed an ability to feel safe certainty as a psychological trick that enables us to live with the knowledge that things go wrong and we are all victims to probability. It is essentially a large part of what makes us human.

As a leader, you likely reached your role based on your skills and knowledge. We often lean on these traits and promote them into contexts, where it serves us again and again. We often fail to see that we are methodologists… we are leaders, teamsters, innovators, problem solvers and entrepreneurs of change. We are not a bag of answers to every situation.

At the peak of uncertainty — when everyone needs an answer including us. The answer is in how we work. We can feel safe with uncertainty, as we can recognise that we are great at thinking a solution out of the air and leading a team of supportive people towards that. We can do this again and again.

When we notice this in ourselves and our teams — the answer ito what is in an unknown future is, "I don't know, but I know how we can get ready for it".

More on this in chapter 9.

Self-compassionate leadership

There is another chapter that addresses this in detail (Chapter 8), so won't repeat here. But realising that you *need* to turn up to soothe your own distress and exhaustion is so very important. When we put ourselves last, we end up being the last one capable of supporting others. A harsh truth in a world of well-intended rescuers and public servants.

Summary

There are many "top tips" to leading through uncertainty and threat, but many of these promote more doing.

Learn how to use stillness and the psychological mindsets that will turn your leadership skills towards being in service of you and not on overdrive in a deluded drive to protect you.

Pause

Reflect

Lead

7. How to leave work at work

Many primary care leaders talk about their work life balance. Working late and taking work home, in terms of stress, rumination, problems and patient experiences.

In this chapter we will share a tool that helps high pressure workers to leave work at work.

The Psychology of Changing Place and State.

Humans evolved from tribal lifestyles into what are now highly complex social, technological and performance environments. The level of pressure and complexity common to primary care staff is a lunar leap from the tribesmen and women we were, despite being only a baby step back in the biological evolution of our species.

Whilst our worlds have exploded in complexity and responsibility, our base biology and psychology is in many ways are much the same as our tribal ancestors. We have been successful in exploiting our psychological resources in creating the world we now occupy.

It is important to pause and think about what life was like for humans pre industrialisation and even pre agriculture. The idea that our brains would be juggling thousands of tasks a day, interacting over digital media, making 100s of complex decisions an hour and all of this embedded in a team of individuals all with similar workloads—it would have been beyond imagination. More likely, it would have made out heads hurt trying to conceive of it! Yet this is how we live and it is *normal* for many of you.

But this is not our entire life. In between these 8–12 hour shifts, we are meant to de-role and return to our lives where we live again like our ancestors—our small tribes (families and friends), with household tasks and social hobbies.

On a rapid daily cycle we are tasked with picking up this complex identity and then putting it down and being emotionally, socially, and perhaps romantically available.

Needless to say, this is a challenge and one that we did not really evolve well for.

We are better equipped to hold stress, ruminate about the day and to take the tension home and release it there at the distress of our tribe, or hold it in until we become ill or isolated, or both.

Punctuating work and home

There is much to be considered about work stress and approach, addressed in this book.

Here I want to introduce a task that helps us to drop work and to become available for our lives outside of work. A task I have taught 100s of professionals and shared with 1,000s of NHS staff via online videos etc.

A debrief.

This is a task that supports us to Psychologically draw a line between work and home—and is surprisingly powerful. I have worked with many terminally ill young men in my NHS role and found this an essential part of my own role, to enable me to arrive home without carrying these experiences. It was taught to me as a trainee clinician and now I present it to you:

The debrief task

1. When work is over, create a symbolic exercise that signals an end. Take off your work badge and put it in a draw. Put your diary or notes in a draw. Take off your work blazer or jacket and replace it with your home jacket. Make this an intentional act in which you are either putting the day in a draw or taking off your 'uniform' and replacing it with your 'true identity'.
2. End work in reality: Laptop and phone off and away until the next day (yes, this can be done—even in primary care!)
3. Journey home: Consciously notice that you are moving away from work and towards home. Consciously invite positive thoughts about home and what it has in it that you love and look forwards to.
4. For remote workers: take a walk and engage in the same task. Create a sense of a commute.
5. Ground: When you arrive home, engage in a grounding exercise. Inform your family that you need 5 minutes to settle in before all of them descend on you—or if you live alone, give yourself 5 minutes before trying to engage in your home life. Undertake an activity that has a sensory component. Take a shower, get changed, drink

tea, light a candle with a smell, hug a teddy… whatever appeals. Breath easily and notice that this sensory sensation is nice and you like it. Notice that it is a sensation common to your home and not work. Invite more of it. Invite yourself home.
6. Arrive home: Now you are home. Work is over. Laptop is away, phone is off and you are present. Enjoy it!
7. (Optional) Panic rescue: Something comes to mind that you realise you need to remember or attend to. Write it down, stick it in your laptop or work diary and promise yourself to get to it as soon as you are 'back' at work. This enables you to let go of it as fear of forgetting often underpins rumination.

Summary

Leaving work is a psychological task but one we can learn.

This task, when practiced daily, becomes powerful on the days when we are most challenged and stressed. We build a practice that can rescue us and always make us available for the recharge that our home lives can bring.

It is not easy, when we are starting from a life where work is not contained—but it is a clear route to changing that.

Put Away

Walk Away

Arrive

8. Four key needs of compassionate leaders

What makes a good leader?

Let's start by asking a question about yourself as a leader,

When you turn up in the room, do your team feel oppressed and observed, or do they feel strengthened and appreciated?

Great leaders are often described as being in service of their teams. The facilitators of others. The enablers of people whose very presence increases the team's sense of ability to succeed.

Beyond the positive experience of this type of leader in a team, evidence suggests that this also underpins the effectiveness of a leader. The main predictor of leadership effectiveness is the ability of a leader to invite, enable and receive feedback from the team (upwards feedback). This being indicative of a leader who is in touch, listening and joined up with the team in their work.

We can name the leadership style that might best facilitate upwards feedback as being 'compassionate leadership'. One definition of compassionate leadership is,

> Compassionate leadership in practice means leaders listening with fascination to those they lead, arriving at a shared (rather than imposed) understanding of the challenges they face, empathising with and caring for them, and then taking action to help or support them.

I can bring to mind leaders of this type, who feel open, receptive, and responsive to the experience of the team. It is a model of leadership I aspire to, and in fact find too easy on occasions—being able to turn up for others and eager to enable my team to meet their challenges as equipped and supported as possible—at a cost to myself.

What strikes me in this definition and in the context of leading during crisis or pressure—is the absence of describing where a leader is compassionate to themselves. Good leadership is very often framed through the lens of behaviours towards the team, without reference to what a leader needs to be present in this way.

This may seem a strange idea to raise to the well-read leader, but I too often meet leaders who are exhausted and stressed, in a role where they are regularly arriving for their team, listening and enabling. These behaviours can inflate to consume the life of a well-meaning leader, who increasingly turns up for the organisation and reduces their presence in their own life and own wellbeing.

What I have witnessed, and experienced is the need to arrive compassionately, for yourself.

Ultimately, the organisation needs the leader to thrive if compassion is to be maintained. As the risk of not doing so is compassion fatigue, and a shift away from being available to just trying to survive your own burn-out. I've been here many times, as have many leaders I support—so this is more than academic… but I've learned a lot along the way.

Self-compassion for the leader—4 key needs

1) Listening with fascination

Being able to hear what is going on for yourself requires active effort, for many people. This means taking the time to listen to your emotions, body and thoughts.

What are you feeling day to day? What is your primary emotional state?

What is your body saying to you? Are you aching? Are you sleeping well? Eating more or less?...

What do you think about and how in control are you of this? Can you think about things beyond work when outside of work?

For many of us, taking a period to sit and write or talk about ourselves is necessary to access this. The same as we'd give to our teams, give to yourself.

2) Understanding the challenge you face

Hearing what you are experiencing is not the same as noticing what you need. The symptom is not the cure.

It is important to recognise that you are a human and you have needs, which may be unmet or challenged. But in this realisation, you need to feel compassionate to yourself. This is central—you may feel stuck or that the current crisis needs you entirely. This may be true, it has been for many nurses and doctors recently, but it is worth being ok with feeling sorry for yourself or wanting to rescue yourself—as you would others.

Letting yourself feel the appropriate compassion for someone in your situation is therapeutic. It's what we give to others when they are in need or distressed.

For many of us, we are even harder on ourselves when times are hard—or if we fail. This lack of compassion to yourself— recognise, it is not how you would act to others and you are as deserving as others to receive it.

3) Empathising and caring

The ability to provide care, as a compassionate leader, is felt by others. We offer ideas, space, solutions, validation, resource.. but we do it from a position of recognising the feeling the other has and caring for them as a valued person and team member. This is felt by others.

Feeling this for yourself.

Recognise, without defence, that things are difficult and the challenge is hard for you. But also recognise that the idea that you have no space for yourself is likely exaggerated by how hard things are. There are always ingredients that can be added to any situation to ease it, but without pause, compassion and intent to provide care—we can be lost in the doing of a situation.

Recognise also that your team need you to care for yourself. A leader should model what a team should do, not just preach. A leader needs to be fit to lead. Compassion needs to be received and not just spent.

Use these realisations to activate a commitment to support yourself, making it reality and not just a lost or distant idea.

4) Supporting yourself

Your wellbeing is the most important asset you have. It enables you to fully turn up for everyone in your life, including yourself. Without it, every role you have will suffer, which in turn, negatively impacts on others.

Consider what you need to have wellbeing and resilience, and this differs for us all.

What pace can you maintain?

What nurtures you, and how can you reconnect with this or add in more?

Who nurtures you, and where are they in your life?

What does your body need?

What do your emotions need?

What does your mind need?

Review all of these regularly.

Need, need, need… it is a word you need to embody as a self-awareness dial. When your needs are being unmet, the needs of those you lead will eventually be unmet too.

Summary

Self-compassion is the foundation of a sustainable compassionate leader. Plan for maintaining this or building this if it feels new. Personally, I regularly fail and succeed at this—but I feel compassionate to myself that this isn't easy.

Pause

Notice

Nurture

9. Embracing safe uncertainty

In the time of most uncertainty and threat, the response seems to be the mass marketing of solutions and answers. Your inbox is likely drowning in offers of certainty, but the future seems no more clear.

Thanks, but no thanks, I prefer safe uncertainty to unsafe certainty.

It is as clear as day to me that nobody has a tried and tested roadmap for thriving through these current times, because they are unparalleled in any chapters of history that resemble our own. The new normal is uncertainty, and it's a feeling we don't like.

I've spent decades supporting people who have had their certainty shaken out of their lives by sudden events. Terminal diagnoses, head injuries, terminally ill children, the sudden death of a family member, violence, war… a common feature has been the realisation that life can swing from planning the new bedroom wallpaper to constant ruminations about finances, death, pain, survival, and recovery.

A normal life can, in an instant, be refocused on threats that feel far from normal—failing to realise that they were always there for us, but we were able not to notice them.

I have found it helpful to be reminded of this reality to live a full life—and to this goal I have a picture on my wall at home that includes a quote from Kierkegaard, it reads:

"Tranquilised with the trivial"

My interpretation of these words is—we walk about in our lives, actively distracting ourselves from the realities of existence at the cost of failing to seize the momentary gift of life.

Don't get me wrong, I love Netflix nights and feel grateful for my ability to engage with the trivial, as it is a necessity for us all.

However, the gift to me of working with people who have been unable to tranquilise themselves, due to what life throws at them, is that I have learned that there is a place for this awareness—and when it can be transformed into a new outlook rather than a fear, it can enrich life and work.

I don't want this piece to drift into being a 'How To' guide—as I am not promising certainty in this chapter. Quite the opposite, I want to invite you to embrace the uncertainty and recognise that you can breathe, eat, sleep and grow with uncertainty just as well as you did before. Except now, you may be more awake and able to notice that life is going on and you are gifted with it.

Let me give a more concrete example…

As I look at now and into the future, thoughts surface.

Will I be affected by COVID in any of the many ways it could land into my life? Will I lose loved ones, lose my income, become unwell myself, see my children ill, experience a worldwide financial depression…? Will our practice survive, will my staff leave, will I maintain wellbeing at work?

Let me tell you.

None of these thoughts ever help and only create pain for us.

No client of mine, with any form of illness, trauma or loss has ever benefited from this framing of an uncertain future. It creates the pain of a reality that we have not yet lived.

Life is fine. You are an expert in living it and in surviving it, that much you have proven.

You just need to realise that uncertainty doesn't mean that things are unsafe. Whatever is coming, I guarantee you that you will eventually feel that it is normal. The internet didn't exist when I was a teenager and yet it feels like it was always a reality.

You have an amazing ability to adapt and to grow.

Breath slowly, accept that we don't know the future—we never did—you are a little more awake now that you notice this uncertainty. Fear can be reframed as anticipation and excitement—feeling alive is truly to feel afraid, as it is time-limited and every minute counts. Don't fear the fear, harvest the energy.

Then play with life and be creative. Whatever way you need to live, only you can work out—and that's something you may get wrong, wrong again.. but eventually right. That's where you are safest— in your willingness to try and accept that we are all just making it up from now on.

Safe and uncertain.

Safe uncertainty

Not unsafe certainty

Go play!

I'll join you there.

(See Chapter 25 for ideas on how to manage uncertainty related anxiety in your team)

Leading Primary Care

"If you find a path with no obstacles, it probably doesn't go anywhere"

Frank A Clark

10. Feeling valued as a practice manager

A primary trait of almost every practice manager I have met is their devotion to their team and their natural inclination to serve.

In my coaching work with practice managers, I have come to realise that the complexity of the role has changed over time. Managers tell me the role has progressed from one of team support and administration, to include rapid innovation implementation, increased governance reporting, managing burnt out teams and the new challenge of the new GP contract and the formation of PCNs.

As a close onlooker, the role is clearly not for the faint hearted.

Many of the managers I meet describe themselves as self-taught. Rarely have any received extensive training in change management, coach leadership, innovation, reporting, team pastoral support, complex network collaborative working etc. Even those with extensive educations in these areas hit the ground and realise that each practice is an evolved beast of its own origin. The core functioning (DNA) of each practice is uniquely different to any other practice—in an environment where individual practice performance seems under constant scrutiny/criticism and it is increasingly difficult to trust others or feel that your back is covered.

The description of the role in its entirety is beyond the scope of this chapter, being uncapturable in any generalisable sense.

Beyond the role itself is the complex dynamic of a practice and/or PCN.

Practice managers find themselves in a complex weave of politics and power, sitting in a business/health service hub where the owners and power (GP partners) also serve as the primary function of the business. In the context of an organisation, this is known as a particularly complex environment to try to effect any changes, never mind rapid and large-scale changes (as are increasingly required from the government and service demand).

Practice managers often find themselves trying to negotiate between a power base that seeks to serve its function—GPs trying to see patients, get home as early as they can to chance to see their kids and avoid burnout or the loss of more peers—and the needs of the rest of the team, the patients, the CQC and the CCG (to name a few).

There is a great deal of chatter about the long hours of work of a GP, but little is said about practice managers.

Most that I meet, at least when I first meet them (as this is an area of need), work long days and are never far from their phones or email. 6am panics to patch up the service with a locum, when a staff member calls in sick, or annual leave email panics when the team has run out of coffee and nobody knows how to order it or who orders it.

Practice managers wear so many hats; parent, shoulder to cry on, captain, inventor, fixer, party organiser, fire fighter…

Yet the question that almost often prompts tears from practice managers I support is, "do you feel valued?".

And in these tears is a signal to a great need for the practices as a whole.

Many times I am told stories of practice partners leaning too heavily on practice managers. Passing on all responsibility but failing to support when asked (often due to their own demands). Needing to be chased to deliver. Expecting the manager to have the answers, to fix the problems, to lead the team—but to not authentically be given the leadership power. Answerable to the GPs, the owners—the function of the business, the least able (in their role) to effect quickly what often needs to be effected.

It's not a power struggle, from my observation. Practice managers regularly communicate to me how they have developed strategies to persuade, seduce, comfort and tiptoe necessary ideas through board meetings. A recent coachee commented,

"as long as they end up believing it was their idea, they will go with it. But I then never take any credit for my work and all the blame when it goes wrong. It is exhausting."

So, how to thrive as a manager in such an environment?

I will offer a brief ideas roadmap towards experiencing value—based on what I have seen coachees work with:

1. Recognise your role and how value is 'felt'

Take time to consider what role you present with the team and what is valuable to you. Many practice managers I meet thrive on rescuing the team and keeping the ship afloat. The list of hats I provided above they recognise well, and perhaps can add more.

It is important to recognise that humans are incredibly poor at recognising a valuable thing or person. The philosopher, Marcel Proust, noticed that when the telephone was first invented, he was in marvel at it as a miraculous wonder and within a very short period of time was enraged if it failed to work. A miracle turned into an annoyance, simply through the passing of time.

We take for granted that which serves us well.

You may have fallen into the category of someone who is essential and a miracle worker but is just unseen—due to the demands that everyone has and the frustration they experience when they need something fixed and are so used to it being smooth, under your leadership.

In this instance, I would invite that you look at the hats you are wearing and try to notice the value you create. You are likely needed… really needed. In truth, it would be harder to replace you than perhaps any other team member—without some serious practice disruption.

Notice this—to be needed is such a great thing in life and does not always need appreciation. We are needed by our pets, children, parents as they age… and rarely do they explicitly appreciate us for our efforts. But we appreciate, in ourselves, that we can give to them.

This is not enough... but is your start... more below:

2. Recognise the system and what is encourages

The NHS is learning to become a compassionate employer. I would argue that it realises this itself. The messages of compassion and support are increasing, in an environment of staff retention and recruitment issues. The work is harder and the team are more in need than ever before.

Recognise this.

You are in a role that is primarily built around serving others and meeting targets, relentlessly. The whole team.

As a leader, your own sense of unity with the team and your own self-development is often put last as you constantly seek to meet the needs of others.

Pause and reflect.

Your team is greater if it is closer and tighter. To achieve this, you need to create the space to lead—and part of that needs your own self-development.

The quickest and most impactful ingredient is time to think, reflect and plan. Lock your door, block the diary, divert the phone for an hour a week and reflect on what is going well, what is needed and how to get it.

Start by valuing yourself and your role as more than just hat swapping.

3. Arrive at leadership and move from management

Leading is a mindset not a job title. Every person in your team can lead in their role and in delivering the value they carry.

Your role invites you to be strategic and to place the team's ability to deliver at the core of your strategy.

To achieve this you need to start passing some of your hats to others and supporting them to grow into their hats. Fixer, party planner, report writer, data gatherer, 6am fire extinguisher… these are all hats you can pass around.

Leading is about enablement of others and yourself.

This may take some work, or even leadership coaching, but is the cornerstone of your ability to access value and to feel valued.

4. Initiate a conversations audit

I have written a separate piece on how to do this, as it is a tool in its own right.

However, for you as the leader of an organisation that needs to feel value—work on how you talk about value and where it is felt.

I can assure you, as I have witnessed through coaching, that many of the GPs feel devalued and a sense that they are on their own. Their own partners seem a million miles away and that they have to keep pushing on.

Learning to enquire about value, to talk about what you value and to invite this as a culture shift is perhaps the best gift your team could give itself.

Learn to strive for this and to brave the conversations needed to get there. It will feel fluffy and odd, in the world of targets and pressure—but the 'soft stuff' is what we all really want and once our egos get past it, we treasure it and it becomes the glue needed to hold a team strong.

Summary

I have the greatest admiration for GP practices and their leaders. Learning to feel a similar admiration between yourself, as a team, and communicating it will be reward in and of itself.

Pause

Expand

Embrace

11. Feeling valued as a partner GP

The role of a GP is intense to say the least.

Most GPs can be considered of as technical experts in the delivery of broad medicine. At the front of the NHS, a GP will meet a vast number of patients and be tasked to make clinical pathway and treatment decisions in a matter of minutes, on loop. To such an extent that I've met GPs who struggle to discuss anything for longer than 3 minutes, the counter to my problem as a Psychologist—being unable to discuss anything in under 60 minutes!

Beyond the role of being a pressured jobbing clinician there are a legion of additional demands including dealing with complaints, medical crisis, personal development, covering for sick colleagues, admin, new technologies, constant change and for many, the ownership and leadership of a small business.

A lot.

But as you will know, many GPs take on additional roles that tap into their special interests, including new clinical skills, leadership and consultancy.

The life of a GP is often packed.

Primary Care teams often perceive GPs as the top of the pile. Owning the business, reaping the profit and holding the power. Of course, this is true—but the culture of the team and how the team feel is not a direct outcome of this, it is an outcome of leadership.

One outcome, which seems not that uncommon, is that GPs can feel undervalued in their own teams. Either through a direct sense that they are isolated or as an outcome of confidence issues in the role of leadership. They can feel unheard, unappreciated, and frustrated. There is no shame in having this need, we all want to feel valued and appreciated for our efforts to some degree.

This is a recipe for problems in practices when this becomes a hidden experience for GPs.

Accessing value

Here I will offer some insights I have learned from supporting GPs towards better connections with their team and a felt sense of value.

Recognise your role and stick to it

Many medics have learned to try hard and to over deliver in the world of healthcare. The system rewards effort and there is a definite culture of presentism—where long shifts and turning up are acknowledged as positive traits.

As a GP, it is important to notice that you no longer have anything to prove, rather you have a business to succeed at leading. Being right is second to being profitable, leading people well and meeting patient needs (which are mutually co-dependent in a business sense).

Being a good GP and having a good business leadership skillset are now priorities and you may need training in the latter. When we feel weak in one area, we lean on the other more. Many a primary care partnership meeting is spent arguing about clinical issues whilst the issues of business and team culture draw less interest or strategic thinking. It is difficult to feel and express value when we are masking our anxieties with ego and dominance.

Learn to invite awareness of weakness in areas of your business and access your most developed skill, being able to learn skills quickly.

Be intentional about value communication

If you can only do one new thing today, communicate value in your practice. At the board level, in meetings and in 1 to 1s— notice value in others and state it. Compliments, appreciation, and verbal reward are fuel to teams. Note that I recommended that you "notice value". Don't look for compliments to give as a team upgrade trick, learn to notice how much you value this tribe of people who have turned up to help you be a success! What a privilege it is to lead those who aid us in our own mission. Connect with this truth.

There is a sub-culture within the NHS, a vocational side effect – where we can often just expect staff to turn up and work hard because that's what we do. Remember though, you own or lead the business and this is a different position than many in your team. Being a positive value spreader is going to encourage the same back. It is surprisingly rewarding to lead on this and you will notice value given creates value back.

Lead a culture that notices value

Build value awareness into your meetings. There is a chapter later on noticing success that I recommend you read (Chapter 23). Teams that can see their successes and where they came from can also build on this to get more of it—in terms of outcomes and feelings. Some of the smallest acts in your practice often go unnoticed and, without you realising, may be the lynchpins of your success. Search for it, name it, congratulate it and ask how you can get more of it.

Recognise others and self as people with needs

It is important to value yourself and to value others in your practice as humans with shared needs. We all need to feel supported across many levels of human.

I met a GP recently who had taken 3 months stress leave after his father died. He told me years later that he was so worried about himself as he was burnt out but could not take sick leave again as his colleagues considered him to have had his "one shot at it" and it would be letting them down.

Avoid this culture. Name it if it is there. Look after each other. The business of leading a business includes listening out for what your team need on a personal level. When this culture exists, it exists for you too. GPs are forged in iron, in terms of personal resilience, or so I am led to believe. In reality, the number of referrals I've had from the spouse of a GP is significantly higher than other professionals I've supported. Spouses reaching out for support that the team are unaware of, as a need, and the GP themselves has parked as none urgent.

Develop an awareness of personal need, team needs and the need of your organisation to be talking about, enquiring about and supporting human needs as a core business function.

See the chapter on conversation audits to help your board to stimulate this culture (Chapter 21).

Train up as a board member

I address this in the 'Navigating the Board' chapter (Chapter 15), but I cannot stress it enough to GPs. If you want to feel valued and to declutter the business by reducing the effect of ego, control and power struggles—train up as a board member / chair. Encourage your colleagues to do the same. The more you can detach from boardroom politics and the often present adolescent antics that sometimes come with untrained boards, the more you will all value each other as professional contributors to a business aimed at success.

The NHS rarely equips you to lead a partnership business, it is ok to accept this and to seek out more learning.

Limit what you give

If you give too much, you will burnout or you will resent those who don't match your contribution.

Give what you want to and feel comfortable limiting what you give to the practice. Balance this with life. Accept a pay reduction if you are giving less than others and you see that what they give is needed. Be sensible.

It isn't all about time and money, it is also about what you commit your energy to. Don't volunteer for all the donkey work or projects nobody wants, learn to say no and learn to commit to what it important. Learn to use the team to collectively solve the challenges of the practice rather than individual volunteers.

All of this is addressed in this book, so read up and make plans.

Summary

Feeling valued is rarely about what others do—it is a reflection of team culture and how we lead, model and engage with it. GPs lead and own the culture, value is within reach.

Own it

Show it

Feel it

12. Spend your time most effectively

In the context of leadership development, I want to draw your attention to your own ability to deliver in your practice, through the concepts of commitments and agreements.

Commitments and agreements

Let's start by considering what is meant by the terms 'commitment' and 'agreement'.

One approach to framing these two words is to consider them as right or left brain approaches to engagement.

The left hemisphere has been associated with rational decision-making processes, where language (our internal dialogue) is used to weigh up or make plans. It is the left hemisphere that accommodates the language centres, for most people, which link to the frontal cortex (decision-making) via our memory centres. The right hemisphere is associated with more creative processes and is considered to be less influenced by language-based arguments, rather visual, emotional and creative concepts.

Left brain processes are more arguably logical or rational (as much as we can be rational) and so work to draw logical conclusions. The logical route to a judgement about a proposed plan, for example, is therefore based on evidence and weighed up arguments, both from others and within one's own internal voice. It seems sensible—so we go with it...why not? However, these 'agreements' to logic are founded on 'facts' and 'argument' that are prone to change or be updated as personal experience is added into the process. They are, by definition, flexible to change and particularly weak when times get tough and pressure builds.

Conversely, right brain processes can be characterised as more emotional and experiential rather than judgement based. When an agreement is experienced as a positive emotional process, such as excitement, inspiration, aspiration etc the agreement becomes more cemented as a goal and is better described as a commitment. These commitments we feel motivated to achieve and so are less influenced by interim negative experiences, such as pressure, failures etc… and so you are more amenable to make repeated attempts, to adapt your approach and to ride the bumps in the road towards something you want.

Commitment Audit

As a leader, it is important to be sure that your work is aligned to your commitments—to yourself, your family and your practice/team. This is not the same as a contract, as it is a wholly internal process—a contract is an agreement. At some point, you need to have consciously made commitments with yourself, the universe, your God… to do whatever it is you are driven to do. Without this, you have no aim in your DNA. No passion to fall back on in times of difficulty and no inspiration to spread to your team.

This commitment is the first step in your leadership career and is often missed or has arrived without notice.

So right now, take time to notice:

- What have you committed yourself to?
- What values does this commitment embody?
- How will you know when you are doing it?

It can help to sit down for 20 minutes and to write these down for yourself. The next internal check-up—which is often hard to not notice if it has arrived—is whether or not you are experiencing wobbles:

- Are you starting to question your role?
- Are you questioning your goals?
- Do you feel unsettled?
- Is there interpersonal drama appearing in the workplace?
- Are you struggling to motivate yourself?
- Do your team feel distant to you or to misunderstand you?

If you answer yes to any of these questions, it is time to re-assess and to update or create your commitment. I would argue that this is central to the function of all leaders. Before you explore other areas such as stress, locus of control, demand, life-balance etc. *(Of course, if your life has significant stress events in it—this may require urgent attention).*

Without a clear idea of what you are committing to, you can't check your agreements and whether or not the context is introducing problems.

Commitment review

At this point, a review process is worthwhile. This is an opportunity to reflect across your work and life to be sure that you are not committed to conflicting goals (between family and work etc), compromising on your values or serving out of date aspirations. Explore the following questions:

- What are you committed to at work?
- What are you committed to in your family / personal relationships?
- What are you committed to for yourself?

Each of these can be broken down using the questions below if you are struggling to connect with your drivers:

- What do you value?
- Where do you experience the most joy?
- Where do you experience the most abundant output, despite little effort?
- What can you do without any external push?
- What does success look like?

(Again, sit down and write this down…. it helps!).

The goal of this exercise is to create clarity, for yourself, about what you are committed to do, achieve and have in your life. Most importantly, these are motivating, exciting and aspirational to you—engaging your whole brain as an emotional and rational commitment.

This is your rudder.

Agreements

As a consequence of this self-development work, the agreements you need to form to serve your needs should flow out of your self-awareness:

- Who: With others who connect to your work, personal life and also to yourself.
- When: as a consequence of your commitments needing to be met.
- What: activities and processes that align with your core principles.

To maintain this flow of agreements—that align with your commitments—you need to watch for any wobbles or drift to old ways of being or organisational norms. The rules are actually quite obvious, but difficult to follow:

- say yes when you want to
- say no when you don't want to (Chapter 13 will teach you how!)
- do what you agreed to do
- don't do what you said you wouldn't do
- work to change or withdraw from any agreements that no longer work for you

Maintenance

As the last point, it is important to recognise that as you grow and your life expands—commitments you make will become outdated. These exercises are the equivalent of engine maintenance—they need to be repeated to maintain the hum of the engine. Outdated commitments will lead to agreements that do not align with your life and work—which could be perceived as external forces getting in your way (stress) rather than recognising that it is time to reflect and rediscover what your life needs you to commit to.

Take an hour every 3–6 months and check your engine is humming.

13. Why and how to say 'no', whilst building cohesive teams

In the context of striving to succeed the dominant narrative is to impress others, be available, network, be helpful and to not let others down. This feels most true for those who lead their own practices, those who are emerging or aspiring leaders and those who want to work in cohesive teams.

When I explore the problem of demand and capacity with practice leaders, which is a common issue raised, I start with an exploration of the commitments that they have made to themselves (see Chapter 12).

From here, we can start to look at the agreements that have been made in their current role to explore where their activity is serving them best and where agreements have filled the diary with work that serves others at a personal/organisational cost.

On face value, agreeing to support the work of others seems like a sensible thing to do to create networks, positive impressions, business leads and/or a cohesive team environment. However, you know that this can also lead to huge pressure and demand to deliver for others that can impact heavily on your ability to be available to meet your own commitments and the agreements that truly matter.

When this audit of agreements reveals issues — like saying yes too often — inevitably, many clients respond with, "I don't seem to be able to say no".

The art of saying 'no'

The art of saying no is more than just a social barrier, it is potentially destructive to morale, productivity, and personal development. I would go so far as to say that an inability to say no is a red flag in a team, requiring support.

A leader who cannot say no is not fully capable of leading to success. In truth, most learn this on their journey upwards — as the ability to focus on their commitments enables them to perform and achieve promotions. Many leadership spotting metrics tease out focus and an ability to deliver on task as valued traits.

Of course, not all leaders emerge in this way — and many are either ambitious to rise or leading as a consequence of building a business and sitting at the top. For these leaders, learning the art of 'no' is imperative.

For the keen team member, an inability to say no can dilute their key role to a more generic role that is driven by agreements rather than a passioned commitment to take the team goal forwards. Agreements with other team members to aid their commitments will water down of their own role, which was likely key to the organisation at some point. In this context, cohesion and team effectiveness requires intelligent delegation and teaming but not heroes in capes. Most team members prefer to be supported towards enablement and rescuing reduces self-enablement of teams over time, so should be avoided.

3 steps to saying 'No'

1. Firstly, you have to really understand where your commitments and key skills fit in the organisation. This is a personal alignment task. What do you bring and how are you emotionally engaged, in respect to what you want and how that aligns with your organisation's mission. If there is no alignment, I'd suggest this needs work or you need a new host organisation. But let's assume there is alignment...

2. Once your reasons for being in this team and role are clear to you, reference this emotional and rational position when asked to do something or feel compelled to rescue a team member. Ask yourself why this task needs you, how it serves your role, how it serves your commitment to yourself (and the organisation) and whether you want to do it. The last question usually reveals the truth if you are aligned with your role and organisation.

3. If there is discord, simply address the situation with empathy and decline:
    - I can see that you are struggling, but I have confidence in you to try and will provide you whatever time you need to give it a go.
    - This is a great opportunity for you to give it a go, as a self-development piece.
    - I'd really like to help and can see that you would benefit, but I really have to focus on my current tasks at present and so I have to say no. Sorry.
    - At present, I am too busy, but I could chat about how you are approaching this over a coffee if you'd like?

- I'm sorry to see that you are stressed, I really wish I could help. I share your experience of stress at the moment with my own tasks and so need to deal with my own work first.

There are many ways you can decline — most of which don't need the word 'no' to actually be stated. Rather, validating the request as being heard, connecting with the need and offering encouragement and/or a reason for your decline. People don't like rejection, but they do like to be heard and to experience compassion. It is the human connection and empathy that creates cohesion — not the requirement to say yes. This is more authentic and doesn't fracture teams, which is a genuine risk of repeated reluctant 'yes' responses.

In summary

The ingredients to saying no are simple:

1. Have clear commitments
2. Check how you feel when asked to help or feeling the need to rescue
   Check if this agreement aligns with your commitments
3. If there are any wobbles — show empathy, compassion, encouragement and decline.

Like all things, this takes practice.
It gets easier.

Just remember — the word yes is not banned, you can help sometimes — when helping is the right thing to do!

14. The skill and psychology of delegation

Following the last two chapters (working out what you need to commit to in your role and learning to say 'no'), it is imperative that as a leader you understand how to activate the support of your team. Saying 'no' to tasks, for leaders, either means that the task is not relevant to your practice or that it is not relevant to your role – the latter implying that it requires delegation.

Delegation is as much a skill as it is a culture within a team and a mindset within a leader.

I hear many practice leaders talking about how difficult it is to let go, to pass on work to others in the team or to pass on the responsibility that goes with the work. Tasks may be passed on, but the anxiety about it being done well remains and micromanagement or similar styles of care taking appear that eventually block great teamwork.

Management skill

Leaders who successfully delegate have usually developed the skills of people management and the psychological safety within the team to be okay with taking a risk.

Delegation is a management skill. Learning how to sit with a member of staff or a team and to enable a staff member to rise up to take on a problem that you need them to solve. Increasingly, coaching skills are trained into managers to encourage staff to seek their own solutions and use their own strengths. Consider this as an approach if your style of management feels directive rather than activating (be honest with yourself!). There are plenty of short courses for managers who want to coach within their style, I have provided such training to practice leaders with great effect.

Managers also need to feel confident in tracking the tasks they delegate out. A project management approach is needed as teams grow and more of the team are delegated to. There are many approaches to this, which I won't try to teach here. But if you fear losing track of tasks and objectives with staff, investigate developing your project management skills and developing a system. At the most basic level, you should be meeting staff regularly as a team and 1 to 1, with your role being to ensure that staff have what they *need* to deliver on what you have delegated. This is not the same as deadline chasing – rather being a servant to your team and using your resource and power to grease the wheels when needed.

Psychological Safety

It is imperative that you learn to sit with the risk and uncertainty of delegation. Staff may well not perform as well as you do with this task and might in fact fail. Consider if your role is to hand hold every task to completion or to raise your team up to function almost entirely without you. If it is the latter, you have to create the space for staff to learn. This means letting them try, letting them fail, encouraging their bravery to try again and celebrating the effort. Failure is learning and when staff are enabled to risk a fail, they risk a win too! When they fear failure, they don't risk and wins become rare.

If you find this too anxiety provoking seek support for yourself as a leader (coaching etc). Lean on colleagues who are more confident with seeing what happens or seek leadership coaching and state this as an explicit need. An anxious manager who fears risk is perhaps the greatest risk to team cohesion and successful delegation. When your own standards get in the way of team experimentation, you are acting as a team of one and blocking the collective power of many.

Delegation

Delegation is a mix of management skill and personal risk taking. When both are blended perfectly, teams rise to the challenge – knowing that their leader has their back and their attempts are celebrated more than the outcomes.

Enable others

Expect failure

Encourage learning

15. Navigating the partnership boardroom

I feel a little like I am walking on eggshells by including a chapter on Primary Care boardrooms. I've witnessed and supported many versions of this, from 2 GP boards through to 27 GP boards and every culture of small business within them.

This chapter considers the psychology of a board and approaches that can support smooth functioning.

A board of clinical leaders plus one.

There is a little-known fact about change in organisations. This being, change is much harder when the leads of an organisation are also the primary function of that organisation.

Put in shorter terms—when the experts are also the boss, they impede change.

This is certainly a risk for Primary Care, where the clinical experts (who also hold clinical responsibility) are also the owners, often the partners <u>and</u> the decision makers. They own businesses that change at rocket speed, with new directives from the government almost hourly and technological innovation demands that assume every practice is full of techno hipsters with nothing else to do than play with new gadgets.

One added complexity, if this wasn't tough enough.

There is usually a practice manager thrown into this mix, often with less power, less income and less ability to make decisions—but all of the accountability for when things go wrong across a raft of variables (income, staff, logistics, bookings, technology etc).

Practice managers are often unsung heroes in the world of Primary care and rarely included in change, innovation, or impact research. This is crazy, as any practice I've known to lose their practice manager suffers a storm of chaos and change whilst an often unassuming newbie tries to catch up at lightning speed with no induction.

Functioning as a board

It is fair to say that leadership training in GP settings is not common. Even when it is, it often focuses on the level of individuals which runs the risk of inflating the power issues stated above or the frustrations of the practice manager with all the skills but no authentic power.

I have witnessed better outcomes when boards develop as a whole and adopt a culture of formal boardroom functioning, that is more akin to other businesses where power need not impede success and change.

I have observed many Primary Care boards operating as collectives, rather than boards. A loose agenda, lots of discussion, very little review, almost no decisions and delegation onto those present or the manager. I have also observed some hefty rows and the use of clinical veto powers to block ideas, something uncommon in many none clinical business boards.

It can be helpful for board members to think of themselves as formal board members and to leave their GP hats outside of board room meetings. Here is simple list to consider for your board, if you don't already, I have developed in my work with boards and often frustrated board members:

- Have a clear Agenda for each meeting which includes a review of previous decisions and actions (against deadlines), agreed points for today and any other business.
- Minute the meetings and all discussions had with decisions made. Send these around and file them ahead of each next meeting. The minutes are the records made by the board on direction, actions and debate. They are, in many businesses, legally required.
- Agree a chair for the board meetings and send them onto board meeting chair training. Respect that they are the chair, as a board—this means that they can stop discussions and reschedule, they can move the meeting along. Welcome this, as it is good for business. Consider rotating the chair if the board prefer.
- Review previous actions agreed. If board members are not delivering on actions, ask for reasons and minute them. Consider delegating away if capacity is the issue or removing the actions. This prevents stalling due to people holding tasks or blocking them.
- Agenda difficult themes with a solution focused commitment, which the chair polices. Name the issue and suggest solutions. Decide. Trial. Review. Try again if needed.

- Clarify the Practice Manager's role in terms of power they have, decisions that they can make alone and areas they lead which the board can vote on but not veto as individuals. Form this as a minuted contract and review quarterly. This empowers practice managers and unburdens the board.
- Delegate responsibility and expect failure. The board is not there to have all of the answers, but to direct a team to solve problems. Don't panic when things go wrong, don't fly in to rescue or knee jerk back to old ways of working. Empower the manager and team to experiment (see chapters 16 and 17).
- Be respectful. Emotions can surface but emotive statements that attack individuals or the team should be policed by the board as a whole. The chair has the power to end interactions and this must be respected, or minuted as infractions of protocol.
- Invite a sense of being in service of the team. Primary Care boards can sometimes feel like the world is on their shoulders and that they are the ones suffering—often airing this in view of the team. Remember, you own the business and you lead it—you can't really complain about a thing you are building to the people in it. It is the team who can complain to you and you need to listen and adapt. Learn to serve the team and they will serve the board through their empowerment. Find a place where you can vent, safely away from those you need to inspire.
- Value each other and make time in the meeting to share this. Compliments are glue for boards! Don't be shy.
- Encourage a culture of noticing what you value in each other and the team and saying it out loud. Boards can be

problem focused but celebrate what you have built together and what it reaps for you, the team and patients. Make this a part of all board meetings.
- Add in a check-in (see chapter 5) to support everyone in getting into the right headspace to be on a board, which can be tough after a day in clinic or putting our team fires.
- Value the practice manager as if they were precious because they are. Practices that lose practice managers rarely benefit (unless the individual was not right for the role), but mostly suffer in my experience.
- Enjoy it. How great it is to be on the board of your own business! Embrace it. Take all the training you can get in leading a board and excel. GPs and Practice Managers are excellent at excelling, but often just assume that leadership is something you can guess. CEOs with entire careers in business leadership take coaching and training… often.

Summary

These ideas are informed by boards that I see work well and the rules are not hard and fast. Be playful with them. If your board feel very fractured, don't be shy—ask for help to fix it! Get a coach or build in reflective space alongside board time. Board fractures get bigger over time, work to repair them as soon as they appear.

Be a board

Act like a board

Embrace it.

Leading Practice Innovation

"Great things in business are never done by one person. They're done by a team of people"

Steve Jobs

"Failure is a part of innovation, perhaps the most important part"

Curt Richardson

16. Innovating under pressure

Primary Care is under pressure to change at a rapid pace – digital innovation, remote working, increased access, digital triage, long term conditions management… the list is mammoth and expanding quickly.

Change nearly always raises fear and resistance in practice teams, at some level. Nobody really likes a change unless the merits of it are obvious and/or desired. This is not always how staff feel about proposed changes, as you know, in practice teams. The reasons for change can feel obscure with teams and leaders talking a lot about innovation fatigue. Constant change is tiring, that cannot be denied.

The NHS is not famous for its ability to change rapidly. There are many references to how good ideas can take 5–7 years to implement across the system. Historically, the system rarely had to change at a large scale in a short time and so its capability to do so is not tested or developed.

Currently, Primary Care is already in the context of staff shortages, staff burnout, unmet demand and increasing pressures to innovate. This has not gone well, with repeated publications relating to the sustainability challenge for Primary Care and the threat of an exodus of staff.

Practices have no choice but to try and change quickly, despite the evidence and obvious barriers to this.

Here we will present some themes that are helpful for change leaders to hold in mind. Many of these might seem obvious, but we cannot assume what is obvious in the context of complexity. They are presented here to validate you as a leader in the face of the need to achieve change beyond what might seem possible, whilst also offering ideas integration into your leadership approach.

Change capability Need

Some ideas to be conscious of when innovating under pressure and at pace:

Pressure does not equal pace.

Simply having a need for fast change does not create fast change, which I am sure you know. The pace of change is dependent on many, many factors and teams are at different stages in relation to this. High resource teams who are already on the path to innovation will change much quicker than low resource teams, with ill staff, long waiting lists and problems within their own teams in terms of leadership. Pressure simply puts further strain on these cracks and can split a team.

The scale of needed change will be pre-set (e.g. online consultation is a whole system revision whereas adding in a new checklist is not), the pace will not. You may feel pressured or directed to change fast but pace is something that is very difficult to speed up past the capability of a team.

It is helpful to recognise that each team will have its own pace and will need bespoke support.

In the context of trying to change quickly, make your culture about witnessing and celebrating your team trying. A culture of innovation is a culture of trying – win or lose. A team can feel motivated to try, fail, learn and repeat on a cycle. This in essence is the ideal of quality improvement in healthcare. How quickly a team is able to repeat this cycle is dependent on the culture of the organisation, where regular feedback enquiries, celebration of effort, collection of team ideas and activation towards a shared goal will increase the pace of change.

Unachievable targets create apathy

Teams need high-performance goals that are both achievable and safe to reach for. When targets are made too difficult to achieve (either by scale or deadline), there is a risk that teams simply detach from trying. Either failing to see any reason to start the impossible or feel that the reason for the change doesn't merit the effort. This creates a real sense that failure is likely, which will reduce a team's willingness to risk the challenge—particularly when they have experienced blame many times over in the media or from patients, for getting it wrong.

Communicating and being visible in supporting the challenge teams face, in relation to pace and the capability of your team, is essential. Getting close to your staff and understanding where their rate limiters are, will be essential to combat a broader sense that your team will either lose or win in this endeavour. Targets need to be set within the capability of your team. This can mean that you breach national targets, but better that than you alienate and lose team engagement. Start early, if your team needs a slower pace.

Buy-in is the key

Change management is dependent on engagement. Teams and leaders need to agree on the goal, the vision and the method of innovation. Engagement is built with a range of variables including the safety for the team to fail and learn, the project goals being compatible with existing systems it needs to fit alongside and the vision of the change connecting with the drivers of the team. When engagement is not there, teams don't work hard to solve problems but see failure or innovation pain as evidence that the solution is a bad fit. No matter the sense of urgency, without engagement from the team (and public), change will not be easy.

Spend time reviewing your team's change progress and articulating the benefits of success. Be willing to accept if it is not returning on these promises and show the team that your practice can adapt and will go with wins and give up on losses.

One size fits all does not create buy-in

At the local level, teams need help to find their reasons to change at pace. This is beyond the national agenda and more attuned to the culture of the team and its journey of innovation in the past. Receptionists may not connect the same understanding of the broader need as GPs and managers, but there are likely shared narratives that can be explored. Rapid change needs whole team buy-in and so this exploration is necessary.

To meet this need, the reasons for change that are on the table need to have adaptability at their core in some part. One size does not fit all—and ownership/adaptability will increase the ability of your team(s) to buy-in. This may need to be restricted to small adaptations, to support scale—but small adaptations are better than no adaptations.

In short – make change a very personalised process that matches the personality of your own practice and listens to the team whilst in action. When it feels like you are pushing your team, pause and consider how you can engage them to be pushing the project and pulling what they need from you. A leader of change facilitates buy-in, points the team and then provides the resources to win.

Attend to the soft stuff!

In the best scenario, practice investment is needed into the people part of change to support success. In the absence of such investment, recognition is needed that teams are being pushed in the worse scenario for change to happen.

Ideally, protected staff time is needed to support the above, the soft stuff… which is in fact the 'hard stuff' for teams.

In our experience, teams benefit when they invest resources into:

- increased visible and accessible project management support in implementation.
- increased change management support that is creative and accessible.

- increased local and regional comms support (for patient and team buy-in), when change impacts on patient experience (e.g. online consultation).
- collaborative spaces for teams to interact (share learning) and debrief (offload stress).

Finally

As the pressure mounts and innovation potentially emerges as the solution, don't blame any part of the system for failing. CCGs might struggle, teams might struggle, individual staff might struggle. Respond to challenge, resistance, defeat, apathy, stress etc., with an open willingness to support and meet need in your own tribe. All of this is to be expected and your practice's approach to change needs to be designed to listen for and then meet the need.

Humans evolved to be curious, to grow, to want to improve… but only when the environment invites and nurtures this. Let's not forget that, even in a crisis.

Ready

Steady

Go (at your best pace)!

17. Winning with large scale innovation

The digital age has brought us amazing technological advances, with undeniable benefit and appeal.

There is great hope that this benefit and appeal will be experienced in healthcare, impacting positively on patient care, staff workload and the overall sustainability of the NHS.

This is yet to be proven.

In the context of no absolute proof, GP practices are now contracted to offer digital-first options to patients in terms of how they access services—with the expectation being that this will expand over time to include new ways of data analysis, healthcare pathway design and even treatment provision.

The largest and most challenging system revision(s) for primary care in living memory.

The response to these expectations is mixed, with pockets of practices embracing the challenge and pushing hard to innovate and implement technology at pace. These are often heralded as flagships for the nation and marketed as a future ideal for all.

The reality for most is that these changes have arrived at the most challenging period for primary care. The sector as a whole is reporting high rates of staff burnout, unmet demand, staff retention/recruitment issues, and low resource. The task of practice managers and partnership boards being primarily about how to meet demand and keep afloat, in the context of what feels like a burning platform.

The question is easy to agree on. How to deliver best practice in this context, without burning out or falling apart?

The solution is less clear.

One solution, now contracted in Primary Care services, is the use of online consultation technologies to support patient access and triaging services—based on the rationale that patient need will be better met with less time spent by high demand clinicians dealing with low complexity issues. The evidence is light that this is achievable, and the sector is aware of this… which has created a range of negative responses for some teams including disinterest, fear, and anger. This is understandable and should not be ignored.

Case example: Online Consultation

Online consultation is not for the faint of heart and I'm a little nervous writing about it due to the mixed emotional responses I get in the real world. It is a whole system revision and requires a shift in working for clinical teams, trusting a remote triage model rather than one that requires person-to-person contact with every patient. It requires changes in clinical practice and the models of access to services—a quality improvement challenge that is complex and beyond what many practices have experienced. There is a lack of trust in this approach, in response to how little evidence there is to suggest that this revision is the solution to the problem.

We regularly meet resistance in teams who are being pushed to implement online consultation. There are shared concerns:

- will uncapped access lead to increased demand, rather than less demand?
- will remote closing create increased risks for patient care?
- will digital triage lead to less opportunity to spot other problems patients have, rather than those reported?
- will access be equal to all patients (e.g. older patients, those with disabilities)?
- will the use of eHubs reduce continuity of care?
- and more…

These are all valid and are in themselves representations of the problems faced, currently, in healthcare access—and arguably on the increase as the age of the population increases and demand on services increases alongside.

Activating team engagement in large scale change

So… how to get past the resistance commonly experienced in teams? Or more helpfully, how to build this resistance into an innovation plan that activates practice buy-in for your team? The answer is in how the change challenge is represented, how your journey towards it is described and what your team agrees to commit to.

For many practices, this requires a big shift in how their partnership boards support innovation.

How to build a learning culture

Here we will describe the implementation of online consultation as an opportunity to build a learning culture within your team—which is justified and needed, independent of whether the technology is the solution or not. The use of online consultation as a case example is intentional, as it is contentious and raises debate in teams and nationally. But this approach is applicable to all innovation in your practice, where large impact will be felt and board culture will be the barrier or facilitator:

1. Create clarity about what the team is signing up to:

Firstly, it is important to realise that a component of the shared challenge for primary care is the fact that large scale innovations are sometimes centrally mandated by NHS England (e.g. Online Consultation both pre-COVID and then with more urgency at the onset of COVID).

This does not always reduce the resistance but is a driver if recognised as such. Resistance now means a larger challenge later when (inevitably) more technology will be coming that needs to plug into innovation successes made today – the solutions themselves and also your practice's approach to innovation, the foundation of future success as innovators.

For your team, you don't have to sign up to the idea that online consultation is the solution—rather that you need a solution to the current challenges and that it is worth experimenting with this one, as you are being contracted to and in many cases the technology is funded by the CCG (true at the time of writing).

The word 'experimenting' is key. Your practice needs to recognise that this is a lengthy trial that will reveal what does and does not work. It is not pass or fail, rather a quality improvement initiative that requires you all to get on board with co-creating a plan, trying it, accepting errors, and learning quickly—a PDSA cycle (Plan Do Study Act).

It may reveal that online consultation does not work for you—or it may reveal that the model for it to work needs a lot of local adaptation and bending around your existing processes (this is most likely, in our experience).

The practice could consider this a 12–24-month learning project—and not look for wins at a fast pace. We have seen many practices take this long to switch telephone supplier! Change is slow.

Learning to learn as an organisation is key—it will enable you to embrace any change challenge, as change is learning and not threat.

2. Recognise the value of teaming up.

Being able to frame an innovation like online consultation as a quality improvement initiative will require your practice to pull together an implementation team that are driving the project forward with the backing of the board, but not the total involvement of the board.

The board needs to agree that this 12–24 month project requires part of the team to deliver and that this sub-team needs some autonomy. This team should reflect the skills and insight needed, so a mix of key people across the practice (project manager, clinical lead, admin, nursing etc). A group who can meet often, to review learning and co-create solutions at pace.

They need clinical oversight, yes—but should not need every decision ratified by the partners board or to have their plans vetoed regularly in response to partner anxieties or resistance. Agreement that this is the plan is the start of this work—the board needs to agree and to see this innovation team as the conduit of feedback in and out of the project, for fast adaption and learning.

The PDSA cycle becomes:

- Plan: the project leader(s) plan the activities into the next period of time.
- Do: these plans become actions through the team—with tracking to be sure everyone does as they agree.
- Study: the innovation team look at the data, feedback and tweak the model with a new plan to solve issues.
- Act: the actions are shown to the partners for oversight and expert input (not for knee jerk responses). If there are no real risks or concerns, the green light is given and the planning restarts.

Beyond your own practice, recognise that shared learning benefits all. So team up with other PCN practices and share what you are learning. Hold a regular virtual meeting or a WhatsApp group just for this—this will reap major returns for all.

3. Crash, don't burn

Most change projects fail. It will fail again and again. This is the route to getting it right for ALL innovation. Don't mistake these fails as indications that the solution is wrong, in the early days—realise that failure is needed to learn.

WD-40, the famous can of spray stuff that seems to loosen off bolts, fix cars etc.. is called WD-40 ('water displacement 40) as this was the 40th chemical composition the company tried before the 'stuff' was effective. 39 fails before a result. Somewhere in their organisation, the leaders accepted 39 fails on the way to success. And it paid off!

Your board should expect things to sometimes feel harder or less tolerable but trust the innovation model to hear their concerns and make adaptations in an effort to fix this. Trust in learning and don't blame the innovation team if things feel wrong. Ask yourselves how many fails are ok, what types of fails are ok and what types of fails are not. Build this into your plan so that the whole team know that failing is fine but fails such as increased risk etc are not—this will reduce resistance as the model will not feel like it has the ability to run wild.

Do not blame any of the team for things going wrong! I can't overstate this. This blame culture will kill innovation—as your team needs to risk failure to find a win. Embrace the effort, accept the fails and strive for the win.

This is the hardest step for partnership boards, I realise. But the most essential. Partners are not always the best people to lead change—they often don't even have the capacity. Being distant to the project can make it feel risky, but this emotional response is not a reason to micromanage and sabotage. The board should reflect on this, with support if needed.

4. Reflect and learn

Take the opportunity, as often as possible, to capture the data that you need to see to assess if you are progressing. Continuity of care, patient experience, staff experience, workloads, QOF income trends… the data will inform the service development.

The board needs to know that this is all being considered, to feel reassured. The practice needs to know what tweaks to the model are steering the outcome towards or away from your overall vision. The innovation team can then justify re-tweaking of the model in the context of this learning, "we are changing X, as we have seen Y and hope to achieve Z".

The practice should want to embrace this as a learning culture—as this is going to be needed long past online consultation. Innovation is the norm for the NHS and the pace is increasing faster than ever seen before. Being a learning team is being fit for change.

Don't shy away from the emotions of team members. Ask for them. Validate if people are disappointed, angry, afraid, etc. This is not an attack on the model, but real team feelings. These are data too and should be valued. When this is noticed and captured—recognised in the ongoing planning and tweaking—the resistance in the team is often much less.

Learning not winning is the guaranteed win

Eventually, you will learn what model of access works for you and what does not work. This learning is valuable, as it will reveal so much more about your processes, pathways and team issues that, if addressed, will better your existing practice setup. The secondary gains out of change management programmes are always huge—as the pressure of change will reveal cracks and gaps that need attention to move forward.

Put succinctly, there are three big wins for your practice if you can embrace this approach to innovation:

1. You will discover what model of online consultation (or any innovation) works for you, in a way that enables your team to get fitter in terms of learning to change quickly.
2. Your team will get additional gains from the learning culture promoted, in terms of understanding why a change programme is hard for you and what you need to attend to.
3. This method will serve you in the future for any innovation challenges or desires you face. This is how change happens best and the better you are at it, the better your team will fare at the level of engagement and capacity.

When learning is the goal, not the implementation success, you really can never fail!

Practices that work in this way describe feeling less pressured, more in contact and more aware of what else they need to work on, which has often been left unattended to for many years.

Try

Fail

Learn to win

18. A game changing skill: process mapping

If there is one skill I'd recommend to Primary Care in the current age rapid of technological innovation and change, it would be process mapping.

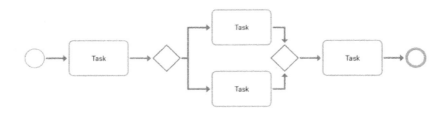

In this chapter, I will attempt to sell you on this idea—getting trained in it or upskilled is relatively easy and there are lots of supporters in the system who can help (AHSN, CCG etc).

Why process mapping?

Process mapping at its most basic is simply a visual representation of what goes on in your practice, wherever activity and people are involved. For example, you could process map:

- your triage model
- your patient flow
- the activities of your admin staff
- the specific roles of a staff member
- the coffee order

In fact, for many practices, the more process maps the better informed the team is and this has a range of advantages:

- The board can see what activity is done by who, when and where.
- New staff can visually see their role and how this interacts with the whole business organisation (especially useful when changing practice managers or lead GPs).
- Proposed changes to process are easy to illustrate to the team.
- Reviews of activity are quick and accessible to all levels of the team.
- Waste in the system can be seen where process mapping reveals dead ends, repeated function etc.
- Current ways of working can be easily compared to new or proposed ways of working in a way that is easy to see and invites conversation or alternatives.

Psychological Benefits

This is a technical skill which brings additional psychological benefits to practices who adopt it:

- Change feels less daunting—visualised team activities and pathways seem smaller and more manageable when represented as pictures on a screen or paper. This invites faster appreciation of a system and allows us to consider change as small changes to an image, with the implications being imagined. This can feel more inviting and more about process than individual ideas of preference or fears about the work involved.

- Team engagement—teams can fear change because the current situation might already feel too complex and not quite managed. Process maps provide a full system perspective of a practice in its parts. This can provide all levels of a team transparent understanding of how their role works in relation to others. This can help staff to feel relevant to the team and to understand why they are asked to do the things they are asked to do, which at times can feel pointless when the whole system is not visible.
- Simulated and experimented change— you can play with process maps and move parts or add parts, then imagine how this might impact on the process map. If data is missing, run a small trial to see what happens then return to the process map to consider if this should continue.
- Co-design becomes more accessible—co-design of your practice with stakeholders (staff and patients) is a gold standard and demonstrated as effective in almost all business settings. Process maps enable this by visualising the way things are and inviting a means to tweak with what might be possible.

Summary

A skill that is critical to complex businesses, which means yours.

Upskill a staff member or yourself, it is as easy as a few YouTube videos and a software purchase.

Or

Invite a primary care project management consultant to support you.

Or

Enquire with your CCG and local AHSN for process mapping support, in relation to new innovations that invite system revision (e.g. online consultation).

It helps if you try to frame process mapping as information empowerment for you, your board and your team. A skill that is so easy to pick up but adds masses of value!

Start

Map

Go

19. Making change happen: the 30-day plan

In many of the chapters of this book there are activities that will raise ideas for future change, at the personal and team level. It is common to see teams arrive at these but not translate them into actual actions. We provide here a simple tool to help leaders and teams to take forward ideas into concrete plans.

This tool, the 30–day-plan, can be conceived of as a simple project management tool—in fact, it is often introduced this way to practices. However, from what I have witnessed, it is rarely offered as a tool to capture needs in relation to wellbeing, culture change and practice success. When it does, it asks questions about individual and team needs—and the organisational requirements necessary to create success.

It is important to realise that when practices arrive at desires to change, even when it is the 'soft stuff' rather than clinical or business related, a project management approach is helpful to cement ideas into the team's intended actions whilst planning for what is needed to achieve them.

30 Day Plan (week 1 sample)

Below is a sample 1 week planner to support your team in taking forwards any change ideas beyond desire and into action (a 30-day plan being 4 weeks). You can draw your own on paper and it is a good skill to learn how to sketch this type of plan out quickly, whenever you are working with a team or individual on any project that needs to be delivered.

TO DO LIST...

30 DAY PLAN
what's achievable?

WEEK 1

what...　　　when...　　　who...

SELF DEVELOPMENT　　*what do I need...*

TEAM　　*what does the team need....*

ORGANISATION　　*what do we need from the leader/ organisation...*

Our quick wins ...

At the end of any team space or reflective session, take time to answer these questions as a collective or alone (respectively):

- What is the clear behaviour or goal the team want to see in the next week?
- When should it happen?
- Who is delivering this?

Beyond this high level understand of what, when and who—ask questions that identify what is needed to facilitate success of this objective.

Identifying personal needs: What do I need or what does the allocated person/people need? Who can provide this and when?

Identifying team needs: Is there something that would benefit you all as a team or is there something that will likely block the team—who can address either?

Organisation: What might the board need to provide or support to enable success. Are there decisions or resources that can be put into place, from the board? What board behaviours, rules or culture might block the team or individual—can this be discussed with the board?

Identifying a quick win that can be achieved this week or month can provide some concrete progress and feel positive especially if you celebrate it with your team.

Involve your team in answering these questions, don't guess. It is this understanding that is key to the success of teams under pressure.

Populate up to 30 days

Repeat this activity across the main team objectives by repeating a version of the example picture given. Either create 4 pages or use a flipchart page and draw 4 columns for each week. Map out projects that the team will be prioritising, making it clear what needs require support and where there may be conflicts or resource issues.

Review weekly and update.

Consider where 90-day plans can help (Optional)

I've seen teams succeed with 90-day plans, especially with large scale change management. Consider this approach.

Summary

It may not seem particularly advanced as an approach, but it is important to observe that the project Gantt chart emerges from this task (deadlines and tasks) alongside the leadership responsibilities that have to occur to enable the team to succeed. It is this latter component that is often missing in project planning or change initiatives.

Consider this a go to tool for any change your organisation needs, for example:

- Implement a new technology
- Advertise a new role in the team
- Upskill the board
- Develop a deputy manager

- Increase the use of compliments in the team
- Arrange a Christmas party

It may sound crazy, but a simple tool can enable staff to feel their needs are noted and the organisation is provided options relating to the impact it has and can have on the success of its team.

Map

Journey

Review

Team Resilience & Wellbeing

"Alone we can do so little. Together we can do so much"

Helen Keller

20. Sourcing team wellbeing from the team.

How do you eat an elephant?

In small pieces!

Alternatively, you give portions of it to a large group of people.

I prefer the latter, although I hope I never need to solve this exact problem.

This metaphor is true for wellbeing also. How do you support wellbeing within your team? You could approach it as an individual need, checking in on every staff member, covering sick leave as it pops up and giving people space to recover, ensuring you have good employment assistant programmes (EAPS) or access to the new NHS wellbeing hubs. All of these, noticeably, are for individuals in need.

But as the government's own report shows – NHS staff are 50% more likely to burnout than the rest of the population at work. There are numerous other studies that show the effects of 1 to 1 staff wellbeing support being very limited, when they return to teams with issues and roles that are overly stressful. This reveals an issue that is in the system, not in the people.

The problem with treating wellbeing as an individual need of staff members is that solutions are reactive not proactive. Staff are fine until they say they aren't, check-ins are looking for signs of cracks forming and investment is made at that point.

Wellbeing is seen as a need for people when they become unwell. It is individualised and placed within the people who need it at an end point, rather than understood as an organisational need at all times, crisis or not.

Team Wellbeing

The word 'being' is interesting as it is both a noun and a verb. I can be described as a well-being (mentally, physically and socially well) or I can be well-being, as in acting well in how I act, feel and think. This is problematic, as I think that most of us consider that we are well unless there are signs that we are not — without the skill needed to monitor, notice, review and adapt. Few of us regard wellbeing as a process of living that may need support when the world around us gets in the way. We have narratives about fighting on, beating disease, but rarely about stopping and accepting that the best you can give to a crisis, sometimes, **is to give to yourself.**

Many primary care teams I've assessed are characterised as being heavily invested in meeting targets and serving the needs of others (patients, staff and the wider system), whilst under investing in personal development and team culture. Giving outwards far more than is given inwards. This is ok for short bursts, but not for sustained periods across the whole organisation. The dangers are obvious when we state this clearly, depletion of energy and eventual disengagement, team dysfunction and individual collapse.

This is simply an unhealthy lifestyle for teams. Similarly, to the advice to eat 5 fruit and vegetables a day, to exercise, to cut down on sugar etc – teams basic wellbeing needs that are not that difficult to meet. When practice leaders are asked how long they think they can sustain this all outwards and little inwards imbalance, many report that they are already failing to sustain.

Your staff crave being in a team

Teams are amazing entities when they work well. I am still amazed at how working with others can not only lighten a task but also transform it into something that refills the tank, when we feel that we are a united pack and in appreciation of each other.

We crave this feeling. Marvel movies, Disney classics and many of the tearjerker stories we are attracted to includes either the witnessing of people turning up to save the day as a collective or people in absence of this and struggling alone. Our hearts leap when a team rise to help the hero and we ache when we watch a lone survivor losing to the odds. Hollywood makes billions by simply showing us stories that tap this emotional need in us, we feed on it by proxy.

I am often told by practice managers, "we can't keep our admin staff as the local supermarket pays more than we do per hour and they get shouted at by patients here".

I tend to ask back, "what did you do to make your admin team know that you absolutely love them for being there for you and that they are critical to your team? What culture did you have that made the admin staff feel like they were as valuable as a GP to your business?". You know when you have done this well, as staff don't leave. This may come down to money in some teams and that may be a fact that needs to be accepted, but more often than not it comes down to team investment of another other kind.

In the non-NHS world, businesses expect to work hard to keep staff engaged. They offer uniforms, discount cards, bonuses, gifts, shares and create an entire company identity that brings the staff in. The NHS benefits from its ability to attract in people who want to do good in the world through public service, but this can lead to the assumption that this is enough in the long-term. We can easily lean on this crutch too much and exhaust people who find it difficult to put themselves first. Sometimes, the organisation must step up and facilitate this for them.

At our evolutionary hearts is the desire to be in a tribe, to be in a team. When we are in teams, even stress and pressure can become an elephant that is broken into pieces. More importantly though, teams bring culture and culture shapes behaviour. When a team culture resonates with care, shared value, safety to take risks, appreciation of all roles and a felt sense of just reward – the behaviours and beliefs emerge to maintain it. These behaviours and beliefs are at their very core a source of wellbeing for the people in these teams.

Creating team wellbeing culture

It is a complicated sell to make to practice leaders and partner GPs, but I've seen it many times over…

When you ringfence the time needed to create the space to think and team up around the biggest problems you have, you create more effective solutions. When you connect the team up as a tribe, you create the protective factors common to functioning families and groups (tribes). When emotions and needs are common meeting topics, team wellbeing becomes an organisational challenge and not the challenge of each individual. When team members feel truly valued, staff retention issues disappear.

This rest of this book provides approaches and ideas that we have seen transform team culture and change the language of team leaders from isolated survival to unity and connectedness.

Join up

Express value

Be a Marvel

21. Essential team conversations.

One of the first observations that I had as a team coach was the great divide between what teams say as a group and what the individuals say, 1 to 1, in coaching.

It is relatively accepted that there are boastful stories and shy stories in all organisations and that these are expressed through many conversations in many places:

- The boardroom conversations.
- The desk conversations.
- The water fountain conversations.
- The afterwork conversations.
- The midnight WhatsApp conversations.

There is a lot being said, by all—in all contexts.

This goes without saying and is a key ingredient of all social environments, the glue that binds people together and the force that divides us. Romance is formed and wars are fought over conversations had and not had.

The value of communication, through conversation, is at the core of almost all teamwork functions. HR, finance, IT, management, clinician, customer, patient. There is no organisational function that can thrive without conversation with others.

As teams form and evolve, subtle and unspoken rules form about what is said and unsaid. A new tribe comes together and the rhythm of its being forms and slowly solidifies into stone.

In our personal lives, we have our own narratives about conversations when we talk about our own families… "we never deal with confrontation in our family", "we never discuss religion", "my parents never mention my Uncle"… this is a common part of family systems and is a commonality to teams also, with one slight difference;

Teams are led towards a mission! (ideally)

Leaders form teams or are given teams, through which a goal is delivered or strived for. A leader has the power to influence the rules and culture of a team, if they have the capability. Leaders can close conversations that are necessary, be unaware that new conversations even exist, or make available channels of conversation that can serve a team and its goals.

Here I will provide an approach to leaders, to audit the conversations that are essential to foster a healthy team dynamic.

Conversations Audit

Ask yourself if any of the conversations listed below, are missing from your own repertoire or your team's?

- Positive enquiry: Are your team encouraged to notice positivity in each other and to express it. Are you telling team members why you appreciate them and prompting the same across your team?

- Failure is expected: Does your leadership include conversations that reassure all of team that failures are expected and the willingness to try is the greatest gift an organisation can ever strive for? Are you encouraging innovation of spirit?
- Try to win: Linked to the above, are you encouraging risk taking to win? Nobody wins from playing it safe—even in healthcare delivery. Risk creates new possibilities and can open the door to new innovations that can bring benefits. Sometimes they don't—but they always don't if they are never risked.
- Uncertainty is the norm: Leaders often expect certainty from a team and this causes teams to freeze. Don't ask for the answer all the time, ask for a display of enthusiasm to work the answer out or fail trying. Embrace uncertainty, as anything else is simply delusional—for all of life is uncertain and it is a failure of the leader not to see this.
- Leaders serve not solve: Do your team realise that you don't have all the answers? Do you even realise it? No individual can compete with a team. Converse about how the team succeeds when they can act without you and serve them to achieve this as often as possible.
- Emotions are allowed: Don't hold back conversations about how people feel, go hunting for them! Constantly lead as a barometer for how your team feel and translate this into action—compassion, support…
- Compassion not blame: Learn to talk about the work of your team through a lens of compassion. Individuals with lives, feelings and problems of their own are helping you

to achieve your goals. Embrace this and allow them to be more than just functions.

Summary

This is not a comprehensive list, but a primer. Rules are easy to break and remould. Create a culture of conversation that allows these themes and guides them in the right direction. Over time, the tribe will learn the new way of being and sitting around the campfire together won't be quite so tense.

Lead

Listen

Converse

22. How much teambuilding time do you need?

When thinking about developing a team building meeting or workshop, the timing is important. In this chapter, we will look at what informs timing design with some tips about where to start for the best opportunity for a team to succeed. Some of the key concepts that underpin this understanding are provided also, to inform your own decision making.

What we know

There is an acceptance in the world of individual change that 50 to 75 minutes is the sweet spot. Therapy and coaching sessions often hover around this period of time, with therapy perhaps having the most robust evidence in terms evaluation – supporting a 50-60 minute session. This is a well-known figure, as many clinical services offer 1-hour sessions and many of us have had experience of theis

In the family therapy world, where groups of people (a family) are supported – there are often two therapists or more and the sessions are typically around 90 minutes. Creating the space for more people to speak, reflect and arrive at some shared growth or ways forwards.

In larger group therapy, where resources allow it, time often flexes around the size of the group. Typical times can be 2 to 3 hours, for larger groups with complex themes. In my own experience, I have worked in 100s of groups / teams where 2 to

2hrs30mins was about the average. In coaching, I've seen groups work together for whole days and in some cases, an entire week (on retreats).

Key considerations in ringfencing the time

It may seem obvious that the time inflates as the number of people increases – but if you ask why, a detailed understanding may be difficult to articulate. This is true for many teams, who may choose to ringfence time together but don't know how much and don't know how best to use the time, if they create lots of it.

To develop as adult humans we need a safe space to think, we need to know how to think (reflection), we need to know what to think about and how to take this thinking forwards into real change.

In therapy (and in 1 to 1 psychological coaching) we support this process through formulation approaches to problem identification and a collective of methods that support reflection, support individual insight and enable real change. This happens at the individual level, in these spaces.

This need does not change when we move into group spaces, as individuals we continue to need this type of support and space to process the team experiences and grow. Therefore, any team building space needs to have space in it for individual thought, paired conversations, reflective work, sharing reflections and arriving at conclusions.

What changes is the impact of a human system, a group, in the same space.

Social groups have enormous power and impact on us as individuals. We can be supported to grow and succeed or be crushed into a corner, by the social environment we occupy.

When groups are together, there is a well-known group effect often referred to by Gestalt Psychologists which states that, "the whole is greater than the sum of its parts". The experience of being in a team and the impact a team can have, is substantially and exponentially larger than that of each individual. This can be true both for negative and positive outcomes, for each individual. Teams can rise us up beyond what we could all achieve individually or push us down and out, dependent on the culture.

It is helpful for us to realise that when the team are brought together and activated in the best ways – the individual problems of staff and the challenges of your practice are potentially dwarfed by a united intent to solve, the recognition of bigger values and successes and the team's collective ability to take on problems as a whole team. It's hard to put into words, but when a team feels connected, we feel at home, valued and eager to support the group. This is the experience we want if our teams are to best function.

Why am I providing this brief 101 class in systems psychology?

Well, really to bring home the idea that organisations ***need*** and ***benefit*** when they invest in ring fencing the time needed for the team to learn how to play together, share feelings, connect, communicate better, and take risks together. Put more succinctly, teams need team building spaces / workshops at regular intervals.

These spaces are characterised by a type of work that is similar to 1 to 1 work, where teams feel brave enough to state issues, learn to explore them together and use reflection to create solutions and plans to change their culture. Essentially, they are the spaces where the culture of your organisation is intentionally designed.

A Sample Workshop for Your Team

It is quite amazing how quickly a team can feel differently, when the right types of spaces are created that invite these types of team experiences. Like 1 to 1 therapy and coaching, a sense of relief and a joined-up desire to change can be felt quickly.

For teams that wish to start this, here are some timing ideas that have come from 2 decades of this work alongside great amounts of evidence about group work design.

Workshop

We recommend a 2 x hour team building meeting, ideally once per month. A sample of what this might include:

- A check-in process to support the team to feel that they have arrived in a fun and safe space (10 mins)
- A positive exercise that supports growth and connections, with individual and team reflection time. (40 mins)

- BREAK (10 mins)
- A challenging exercise that lets the team practice dealing with the prickly culture issues, again with individual and team reflection. (40 mins)
- A summary in which the team arrive at agreed actions to experiment with, to change the team culture. (15 mins)
- Rapid check-out to support the team in naming their experience of the process (5 mins) and celebrating how appreciative you are of each other for turning up for the team.

This is adequate for teams of 5 to 15 people. Any longer and we have seen teams fatigue very quickly, any less and you lose some of the key ingredients. Of course, teams vary and you can follow your instincts. But this is a good place to start and will provide insight into whether your team wants more, less or has arrived at its sweet spot.

Summary

In our work, when time is precious and teams are stretched – I prescribe no less than a 2 hour meeting once per month. This is an investment of 30 mins per week into the running of your team as a group who feel good, get a lot done and resonate union.

When struggling team leads tell us, "we don't have time for this" I don't compromise, as our evidence shows that any less time spent on the team culture is the surest way of communicating that there isn't a team, just individuals working in the same place. The most common testimonial we receive back is how valuable teams found this time once secured and how committed they are to keeping it.

Investing into team functioning is critical for many teams. I've seen many times the impact of how spending this time buys time through the improved working of teams, but it is a leap of faith for many practice leads to take. The question to ask, in all seriousness, is can your practice afford not to? Less seriously, leading a team that feels connected and positive is a delight and makes your work feel a whole lot better.

Our work shows improved engagement, retention of staff, confidence, team connections and reduced stress over the team. All for the low, low cost of 2 hours per month.

Ringfence time

Play

Create capacity

23. Four steps to increase your practice successes

When teams meet to discuss challenge or to work on their own team development, there is a risk that the language can feel problem focused. We all have experiences of teams stating out loud themes of need such as,

- we need to communicate better around difficult topics
- we need to be less critical
- we need to speak up more
- we need to get more ideas from the team
- we need to give a voice to all of us
- we need to meet less
- we need to meet more

Where teams are sometimes great at identifying problems, they can regularly struggle to redesign culture and behaviours towards team growth. The past is often the best predictor of the future - teams often rely on what they have tried before to create change. This creates circularities, as we see groups use the same methods to try to create something new. It can be helpful for teams to recognise that what got us to this point, does not always help us to get to a desired new point.

This isn't to say that teams do not have the internal insight and wisdom to achieve change, more that teams often rely on the same methods in trying to access this insight and translate it into change. This includes the way teams talk about problems and solutions.

This is where appreciative enquiry can help.

In this context, it can be helpful to think of appreciative enquiry as a communication tool that can help teams to dig deep into what works well in the team (even if it is a deeply hidden gem and rarely seen) and then to activate team interest in making this more common for the team. This being an action plan rather than a list of challenges or needs.

Appreciative Enquiry Exercise

Here is an exercise to help a team through this:

Step 1: In pairs, interview each other two questions (5-10 minutes each, rotating roles):

> 1. What have been the most rewarding/valued experiences in your time within the organisation (or team)?
>
> 2. What were the conditions that made the experience possible?

Step 2: In groups of four (joining up 2 pairs) enter into a discussion (20 minutes in total):

1. Share your insights from Step 1.
2. Identify 1 to 2 of these experiences you'd like the team to prioritise as something they want more of. (Don't worry, the team can return to this exercise later to address the others).

3. Answer the question: If those experiences were to become the norm, how would the team have to change?

Step 3: Discuss as a whole team (20-30 minutes)

1. Which 1-2 experiences do the whole team feel should be magnified as a priority for the team?
2. What changes would the team need to make?
3. What actions will each team member commit to, to shift the dial 5% towards making this real for everyone (actually write these down for the whole team and also individuals plan this into their work calendar).

Step 4: Review in the next team development meeting (10 mins)

1. Discuss as a team what happened when you tried to shift the dial.
2. Ask what new commitments individuals might need to make to shift the dial.

Repeat and make a common component of team development.

Bitesize Version

This approach can be incorporated as a smaller approach into team check-ins. Asking the team to notice what has gone well, what they are most proud of - and to expand with a "how did you/we do this" question. Creating a culture of repetitive enquiry into success can change the experience of a meeting space and the direction of future problem solving. We'd still advise a deeper dive with the exercise above at intervals, it is designed to tap the introvert or quieter diversity in the team - check-ins run a risk of giving voice to boastful stories and not the shy stories that may hold the real gems! See our chapter on check-ins for more detail on their value, if you don't do this already (linked below)

Summary

We've seen this work with teams many times over. It is aimed to be fun and positive in focus. Don't be afraid to repeat the whole exercise as often as you need to and consider this an opportunity to play, listen and learn about your team. The team are aiming for better and should see any challenges to this as an opportunity to be creative.

Appreciate

Invite More

Learn

24. Check-ins and why they are an obvious must

The world of work, for many practice leaders, can be experienced as a whirlwind of meetings. Meeting with partners, patients, commissioners, reps and of course the team itself.

It is important to recognise that whilst this is what 21st Century work looks like, it is a far stretch from how humans evolved culturally, socially and psychologically. We are tribal by nature and our psychology has learned to adapt to this new mode of operations - where we can be in new tribes by the hour and on the hour - often with no time in between. We can also, more recently, expect for these spaces to be digital and so a further step away from what we have evolved to accommodate. Now, we face a screen full of faces all looking at us at once - minus much of human non-verbal communication and often with our own face looking back at us too!

Check-ins

When working with teams, groups and clients we have been trained as clinicians to utilise the check-in process. Some examples of check-ins, to be clear about what I am referring to. These exercises being the initial component of a team meeting for all members to be included:

- each stating how they are feeling right now
- each stating what they are bringing from their workday / week that is perhaps difficult to let go of

- each stating what they hope to achieve or expect from the meeting today
- each stating what they have experienced about the team this week, that was positive
- each stating what their energy level is like, out of 10, ahead of this meeting

We train teams in this approach too, as the benefits are often more than might be expected:

#1: Transitioning Spaces

Whatever we have come to accept as normative now, we are physical beings in a physical world. For millennia, we have moved between spaces and our psychological frame shifts and adapts as we move. When we are in a bar we have a different role, expectations and social script to when we are in a meeting with our colleagues to when we are in our dining room with our families.

The world of work requires us to often shift out frame of psychology in an instant. Perhaps moving from a planning meeting into a sales meeting, or a management meeting into a crisis solution meeting... We can experience these back-to-back, the whole day - no wonder we get tired!

The problem for teams arises when teams meet to develop the team or to invite innovation. In these spaces the team needs to be able to access playfulness, creativity, trust and all of the other good emotions teams can bring. This can be very difficult when we don't have the signal we have evolved to need, to signal to us that we have moved to a playful space. We are perhaps still using Teams, in the same room, or entering the same board room we had a stressful meeting in 2 hours ago. Our minds have not had a prompt that this space is for something very different - and so it can rely upon associations and take shortcuts to put us in a state of mind and emotion.

This can mean that teams arrive together with emotional states and expectations that are very out of sync with a team development goal.

Stating out loud what the meeting is hoping to achieve and then letting the team state how they feel in relation to this goal can be helpful. Team members get to notice where they are in relation to where the team needs them to be and the team gets a barometer on how much it might need to support team members in arriving psychologically.

#2 Mental Health Awareness

Asking each other to state how you feel and making this a permissible act within teams is a valuable approach towards creating team understanding, compassion and an overall awareness of individual and team need. The team, and leaders, can observe if there are general feelings common to the team or repeated feelings common to individuals. This creates a broader sense of team or individual need, beyond the goals of the organisation. Inviting and permitting emotions to be stated is powerful for teams and should be practiced. Quite often we hear individuals state that emotions should not be brought to work, denying that we do even if we don't want to. When teams model the disclosure of emotions, it breaks down barriers and shows team members that this is a safe topic.

#3 Acceptance of difference

Observing the two points above, it is an expectation that team members will not always feel the same or embody the same energy or engagement, at work. This is not to say that team members are letting the team down if they feel disengaged or tired.

When we hear the difference between team members, it affords the team the ability to understand why a team member may not be forthcoming, may be overly critical or maybe disinterested in a theme. When we understand the inner worlds of people, we avoid making the wrong interpretations of their actions. For teams this is critical, as many of us personalise the behaviour of others and this can create cracks in teams. If a team member seems disinterested - we can feel that they feel that we are not capable, or they dismiss our ideas etc, etc... but when we know that they are tired and distracted, we can account for their behaviour.

This may seem like it is not rocket science for you, but across a whole team the risk of misinterpretation is magnified.

When we hear how the team members are in this moment, we can acknowledge the challenges some team members are experiencing and continue the meeting. It is a surprising outcome that when people feel heard and have spoken, they can shift in themselves to join the team that is being supportive.

#4 Containment

When people try to hold in their experiences - be these thoughts or feelings - the outcome is that they tend to spill out in other places.

When we invite check-ins, we invite the sharing of experience and challenge into a supportive space. We are creating a safe space to state what the current issues are. We are NOT inviting team members to attack / blame each other or the team, but to simply state what they are feeling or thinking that may be a hinderance to working well together today in this space.

This can be containing for people. When they realise that the group can hear and hold their challenges, without rejection, panic or desperate attempts to rescue - it invites more sharing and more group communication.

Sharing of experience into safe spaces is the bedrock of all therapy and at a less intense level, is useful for all groups of people in a similar fashion.

Safety for a team is the team hearing, showing compassion and then moving forwards with this compassion in mind. Leaders can pick up 1 to 1 on any themes that sound like they need support, for the team, it is enough to be able to hear each other.

#5 Connections

Check-ins can be littered with positive communication. Beyond sharing current place and state in the language of challenge, we can also share this in the language of appreciation and value. We can talk about what the team has achieved, how it has helped us individually and what we value about it or members in it.

I have seen many teams shed tears when they talk about why they want to be in the team and what they value. These conversations are important to have on a regular basis and can be activated as very brief check-ins. Recognise that in the world, when we want to connect with people, we are intently positive about our experience of them.

Summary

Check-ins are often more than teams and leaders consider they might be. They are worth playing with in team spaces, so give it a shot if you haven't already!

Ask

Say

Hear

25. Energising and leading an exhausted or disengaged team

The energy of many practice teams has depleted.

The energy of leaders, like yourself, is likely low too.

Leaders have a role in practices, to lead teams through fatigue and towards a culture and relationship with work that promotes energy, enthusiasm and engagement. Here are some ideas we've seen team leaders in many settings use to great effect:

It is okay not to know the answer.

It is okay to say, "I don't know" to your team, when questions are asked about the future. Modelling certainty can lead to proving that you are wrong or put pressure on you to be right. Teams often feel anxious but it can be validating for them to hear that this is a shared experience.

Encourage 'teaming'

Rather than offering solutions to unknowns, remind the team that you have confidence in them to solve the unknowns collectively. Invite them all to offer ideas and solutions, for a collective idea about what might be the answer.

Encourage errors

The team don't need to get it right every time, they just need to be good enough. This means that you, as the leader, lean on them to lead trials of ideas and to join together around learning from them as you progress.

Find wins

Find reasons to celebrate as a team. When you try something—celebrate. When it fails—celebrate what you learned. Don't go overboard to the point of patronising, but do authentically share your appreciation of a team who are helping you to be successful as a leader.

Have short term goals

Make sure that short term goals are easy to get to and that you notice when the team get there. Communicate them frequently.

Have a vision

Keep a long-term vision. This helps people to realise that you trust the organisation to survive and for the future to be less about current gripes/pains and more about business as usual. Be sure to openly communicate your vision in team spaces, to help all team members to get their own focus off immediate fears and future ambitions.

Enable don't save

Work towards hearing what the team need to succeed and support this. Ask team members to check-in emotionally so that you can hear how your team feel. Make this a human enquiry, not a survey. Don't try to save your team from their own distress. Rather, hear what they feel and keep this in mind as you interact. Offer people what they might need to succeed.

Notice people

Work hard to see what people are doing each day. Maybe introduce a 'man of the match' approach, where you spot something in your team each day and reward a member of staff for all to see on the excellent contribution they made. This can be small, the way they handled a client or the way they cheered the team-up. Create a culture of noticing and rewarding.

Communicate energy

Lead meetings with positive language and a forward-thinking style. You may be exhausted and fearful, but you need to manage this in your own leadership spaces or coaching. Do not project this at the people you need to activate to enable your success.

Be compassionate to them and you

It is fine if your team feel low or anxious and tired. Many of us do. This is likely a normative response to being locked in. Be able to hear it, empathise and then move on towards encouraging success at work, with your support.

This is true for yourself too! I have written about self-compassionate as a leader in a previous chapter.

Redirect firefighting topics to solutions

Responding to crisis and pressure conversations with queries about how to get a solution is an effective route. We've used this approach with over 1,000 NHS staff and have evidence to show it works. Find out what your team think, how they might be able to solve problems, what they need from you to get the problem solved, what it will look like when it is solved and who can start off with solving it.

Summary

Teams are an amazing resource when activated and energised. As a practice leader, you can play with your own approach to support this for your teams. This doesn't mean you have to be full of energy. It means that you support a culture that authentically believes in a future when everything will be okay and is aiming itself at that—despite the pressures of today.

Breath

Think Solutions

Lead.

26. Create capacity through team optimisation

One of the most significant barriers experienced by teams is the experience of not having enough time. This was problematic pre-COVID but seems to be what was referred to as the 'new norm' since the world has resurfaced.

In this chapter, we will look at the reality and psychology of 'not having enough time' and touch on some counter concepts that teams can find very helpful.

Time at work

The idea of time in the workplace is an interesting one, psychologically.

Humans tend to be myopic – we tend to struggle to keep the big picture, the long-term view in our perspective. This is exaggerated when we are stressed, tired or experiencing sustained pressure.

Time shrinks.

Not only does time shrink, but so does our ability to think beyond our usual solutions and ways of working. We tend to isolate, work in a tunnel vision fashion, and innovate less.

This is perhaps best summed up by the words, "firefighting". A phrase we hear often from practice leaders under pressure with mounting work. The role becomes close quarters fighting against fires that pop up here and there, problems that are immediate and small – in a context where the embers seem to be carrying off and sparking new fires at a rate that ceases progress beyond this activity.

Firefighting is exhausting and does not feel rewarding as a work function.

When teams and staff are tired or burnt out, we regularly see staff experience their role as firefighting. Typical tasks start to feel more like problems, other staff members feel like problems, the role feels like it is stagnating, and the job can feel like survival more than progress. It is interesting to connect the words firefighting to burnt out, both making reference to fire and revealing that only so much of this can be sustained before we ourselves succumb to the flames.

In this space, working harder and more hours is counterproductive. Yet it is often the approach taken by team leads and teams. We are raised on the idea that working hard equals more success. We transfer this over to the idea that problems can be solved in the same way. Teams chase targets, leaders chase teams and success is the experience of getting another fire put out.

It is at this point that we are often called in and we practice team leaders. They ask us for help, and we introduce our ideas and services. Almost always, and I do not exaggerate here, we hear back… "but we don't have the time to do that".

We don't have time

The phrase "we don't have enough time" is in fact the next pandemic. It is so common from teams we meet, that we title our programmes – for teams "without any time".

The first step for team leaders is to realise that time is not the problem, it is what we use time on that is the issue. This is not meant to be patronising, bear with me.

When I meet a team, I ask… "in making the statement that you do not have enough time, can you also reassure me that your team feel valued, feel united in solving all of the problems, feel like they are each being utilised the best way they can be in terms of their own skills, feel in control of their part of the team mission and (perhaps most importantly) truly feel that what they are doing is needed by the team to feel successful?"

A long question.

What happens when you ask this of your own team?

When teams do feel valued, well, collectively problem solving, best utilised, on board with the mission and deeply connected to their part of the mission… they work smarter.

Working Smarter

Working smarter simply means bringing the team mind to issues, rather than individuals and fractured thinking. Recognising that big things are made small when we break into manageable pieces. Also recognising that the whole is greater than the sum of its parts... put another way... a united team is FAR more productive than the same collection of individuals working in the same space, independently.

Pulling a team together – in terms of how they feel together – and what this creates in respect of behaviours, is the best way to create capacity.

It feels counterintuitive to tell team leaders to slow down and to ringfence time to get the team to like working together. To notice what they feel. To want the mission to succeed. To want their role to shine.

Teams can achieve this in 2 hours a month! Not a made-up number, but a number we have researched and proven time and again with teams (see chapter 22). We've delivered workshops that harness this team spirit almost immediately, with core components including:

- Using check-ins to create playfulness and team safety (see chapter 24)
- Conversation audits (see chapter 21)
- Appreciative enquiry (see chapter 23)
- Coaching conversation training for the whole team.
- Culture design work (see chapter 21)
- Values identification
- Rapid mission statement creation
- And more...

Many of these approaches can be researched by teams and played with together.

Our advice to teams who want to try something new is simple:

- Ringfence 2 hours a month minimum (see chapter 22).
- Add a check-in to state that the meeting is playtime for the team and not work time (see chapter 24).
- Spend time getting to know each other in this space through conversations and play – not about work (see chapter 23).
- Celebrate that you turned up to do this.

Seems small, but the connections are the glue that make the rest possible.

We are yet to meet a team who don't keep these spaces once they have successfully created them!

Have faith

Leap

Team up

Summary

Leading primary care is a complex and challenging role for managers and GPs. It can be a source of intrinsic and extrinsic reward, but also a place where feelings of challenge, pressure, stress, underappreciation, and team dysfunction can emerge despite everyone's best efforts.

The ideas in this book are hopefully accessible and promote thinking and planning that might create sparks of energy and connection in you as a leader and your collective team.

Don't be afraid to seek help whether it is training, coaching, team interventions if you feel that capacity and challenge are too obstructive. These support services exist for a reason and are readily accessed by businesses of all scales, to get through challenge. Healthcare work has a culture of working more to get to the other side which can be difficult to break out of.

I encourage you to be playful. A strange word perhaps in a context that seems so very critical to the nation. Playfulness is simply the state of being that allows you to chance that an idea might work and to play lightly with the results and approaches that enable you to adapt it to your own team.

Teaming up to enable patient care

I use the phrase "teaming up to enable patient care" as it is perhaps a good mission statement for Primary Care teams. *Public service* captures very well what I see in practices, aiming out at the public and being in service at almost any cost. What is missing in this work category is the team and its culture. Teaming up is a powerful phrase, as it embodies connectedness, unity, shared values and a mission. You might want to consider your own mission that puts your team wellbeing alongside your outputs.

Working in service of your team you can enable them to reach for the stars.

Arriving as the leader

Working in service of your own needs, you can realise how important this is for you and for your team.

This includes being aware of what you need, balancing work and life, learning to develop as a leader in the areas you fear most, embracing safe uncertainty and being compassionate in the face of regular failures and losses.

Primary Care leaders are of so much value to the rest of us, as patients. Looking after yourself is a priority for us, even if many of us don't realise it. It is a priority for you, in terms of your own responsibilities to yourself. It is a priority to your team, who would face a storm if you collapsed from your role.

Beyond being sustainable, learning to use your role to activate your team is perhaps the most rewarding experience a leader can achieve. Lean into this idea and play. Invite your team to teach you how to do it better.

Going forwards

These ideas are not an entire solution, and many may not fit your team or desired culture. They are a nudge towards reflecting on new ideas. Explore in every place where new ideas might appear, asking what might improve your resilience, your leadership ability and the experience of your team in your presence.

Work hard

Play lightly

About the Author

Craig Newman is a Clinical Psychologist, behavioural economist and qualified coach, with 2 decades of NHS service and experience. He is the CEO of aimyourteam.com, which provides support services to public sector teams, predominantly Primary Care. In addition, he founded 'Project5.org' which is a free wellbeing non-profit supporting NHS staff experiencing burnout.

Through the organisations he leads, he has have facilitated the training of over 1,000 wellbeing practitioners, 1 to 1 wellbeing support for 1,000s of NHS staff and has directly developed national and regional programmes of innovation and wellbeing support for NHS services including Primary Care alongside coaching teams and leaders.

His services for Primary Care are designed specifically around the research he has led and continues to lead in this space. This includes specialist support programmes for practice managers, GPs, admin staff and whole teams. Aim your team also hosts the first digital team coaching programme specifically designed for primary care teams, enabling teams to access coaching in a flexible and affordable manner.

For more information, visit www.aimyourteam.com.

Printed in Great Britain
by Amazon